Second Edition / Completely Revised

Guaranteed Potency Herbs

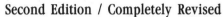

Next Generation Herbal Medicine

Daniel B. Mowrey, Ph.D.

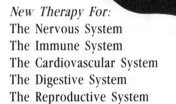

New Therapy For:
The Nervous System
The Immune System
The Cardiovascular System
The Digestive System
The Reproductive System

Milk Thistle
Ginkgo biloba
Bilberry Centella
Butcher's Broom
Ginseng Echinacea
Turmeric and more

Keats Publishing, Inc. New Canaan, Connecticut

IMPORTANT! The information contained in this book is intended for educational purposes only. It is not provided in order to diagnose, prescribe, or treat any disease, illness, or injury. The author, publisher, printer, and distributor(s) accept no responsibility for such use. Those individuals suffering from any disease, illness or injury should consult with their physician. It is hoped that the education of the public about the principles of alternative medicine will lead to a more widespread acceptance of those principles by orthodox medicine with the result that a greater degree of validation and acceptance will ensue.

useful
disclaimer

This book is dedicated to all those herbophiles
who read and expressed appreciation for
their worn and battered copies of
The Scientific Validation of Herbal Medicine.
Keep up the good fight for knowledge of wisdom.

"In your explorations of the realms of science, for undiscovered truths, and unknown and untried agents, seek not for potent poisons, but stop and examine the simple plant under your feet; for in it wonderful curative properties may be found."
L. Stanton, M.D. & D.E. Smith, M.D. *Presented at the Annual Meeting of the Eclectic Medical Society, June 12, 1867.*

NEXT GENERATION HERBAL MEDICINE

Originally published by Cormorant Books 1988. Revised edition published by Keats Publishing, Inc. by arrangement with the author, 1990. Copyright © 1988, 1990 by Daniel B. Mowrey.

Printed in the United States of America

Published by Keats Publishing, Inc.
27 Pine Street (Box 876)
New Canaan, Connecticut 06840

Table of Contents

1

Preface

1988

Since the publication of the first edition of this book, there have been large strides made in the effort to introduce Guaranteed Potency herbs to the American marketplace. More and more American manufacturers have begun importing these herbs and introducing them to their lines. For the most part, this effort has been going forward honestly and carefully. I am personally aware of just a few instances in which the term "Guaranteed Potency" (or a similar term such as "certified", "warranted", or "assured" potency) has been flagrantly missapplied.

The reader should continue to keep in mind the important distinction between standardized extracts and guaranteed potency herbs. The first case involves herbs in which the **presence** of certain constituents is guaranteed, usually in some specified amount. In the second case, both the presence and the **potency** of certain standardized constituents are guaranteed. Potency refers to both safety and efficacy or effectiveness.

The term standardization is problematic. First, there are no standards. What kind of standard is it, when one company's standards are different from another company's standards? At this point, some companies will not even share their standards with other manufacturers. In this country we desparately need to reach some sort of mutual aggreement among herbal manufacturers about standards for herbal preparations. We lag far behind Europe in this respect. Standardization is the first step toward Guaranteed Potency.

The second problem with the term standardization is that it just refers to **technology**. Standardization only involves certain chemical and mechanical procedures to produce a given product. As the technology improves, products of greater purity and uniformity are achieved. Brewing a tea represents one end, the crude end, of the technology continuum, and liquid, concentrated and freeze dried extracts are examples of the high tech end of the continuum. But nowhere in the standardization process are **scientific** studies conducted. It is just assumed that the manufacturer knows beforehand which constituents are active — which constituents are worthy of standardization. To be sure, these guesses are usually based on *previous scientific* work. But sometimes such guesses are wrong, and critics of the standardization technology are correct in pointing out that industrial manipulation of plant materials can destroy important interactions among constituents, change the overall safety profile of the herb, and otherwise louse up what Mother Nature so nicely provided. The only worthy response to such criticism is controlled research: science. This is a costly and time-consuming approach to herbal medicine. Are the end-results worth the effort? I believe in the case of the herbs discussed in this book that the results have been well worth the effort.

What science has achieved during the past 20-30 years is to validate the safety and efficacy (guarantee the potency) of several standardized herbal products that are much more effective than the raw materials. The process normally goes like this:

raw material
▼
standarization of certain constituents
▼
research of safety and efficacy
▼
further refinement
▼
further research on safety and efficacy
▼
further repetition of refinement and research
▼
end product with increased safety and efficacy

A Guaranteed Potency herb, then, is one in which technology and science have been wedded in a product that is medicinally superior, and perhaps safer to use, than the original plant material. For example, raw unprocessed ginkgo is virtually unusable for treating seniltiy, but in a concentrated, purified form, it is one of the best agents currently available. Ingesting enough leaf to produced the same medicinal action would be accompanied by severe side effects, but in the Guaranteed Potency form, side effects are minimal.

Since both the technology and the science of modern herbalism are relatively new, you can find variations and gradations on the main theme. Not all herbs are suitable for the guaranteed potency approach, but the efficacy of all herbal preparations can and should be subjected to validation. Standardization is a prerequisite of validation, which is a prerequisite of scientific acceptance. Without standardization, valid science cannot be accomplished. Imagine the problems in having plant material rich in active principles in one study, and devoid of activity in the next. With reasonable attention to safety, we can enjoy standardized herbs, and profits can be used to further scientific validation in the meantime.

Daniel B. Mowrey, Ph.D.   *January, 1990*

4

Part One: The Herbs

I. Introduction.

The Awakening.

During the past decade or so we have witnessed a phenomenal rise in the popularity of herbal medicine in America. Recovering from the medical/technology revolution that came infinitely close to completely destroying folk medicine, we have been in the process of rediscovering our medical roots, and we are finding that they aren't all that bad.

Part of the American reawakening has been the discovery that our European and Asian counterparts have not slept nearly as long nor nearly as sound. When I first began collecting scientific information on herbs, I was impressed by the quantity of data that had accumulated overseas. There was perhaps only a handful of people in the United States even aware that such data existed. And no serious effort had been made to impart that knowledge to the public. Since the publication of **The Scientific Validation of Herbal Medicine**, I have noticed an increasingly greater degree of public sophistication concerning herbal medicine in the United States.

Catch-Up.

And so Americans have been playing catch-up with the rest of the modern world. Our strides have been long and strong; the gap is closing. But Europeans have not been resting on their laurels. Recent developments in the European market can only be described as revolutionary. A revolution involves a change in the basic ways in which we view a subject. In this case, we have been forced to discard an almost universally accepted theoretical limitation on the potency of herbal preparations: A fundamental proposition of the past had been that any given herbal preparation was limited in effectiveness by several factors: 1) growing conditions, including soil, fertilization and insect control; 2) climatic conditions, such as rainfall and temperature; 3) harvesting procedures, including when and how; 4) curing

5

procedures; 5) processing and preparation methods; 6) packaging; 7) storage; and 8) shelf life.

Guaranteed Potency Herbs.

European researchers discovered that most if not all of the variables listed above could be artificially controlled if you could standardize the amount of active principle in the final product. Then it wouldn't matter if it took one bushel or 100 bushels of raw material — the end product would be the same. There were two hitches: knowing the active constituents of the plant, and being able to measure their presence in both the raw and final product. Actually, there was a third hitch, standardizing the product, but that could be worked out while the basic research on the first two took place.

Efforts to solve the two main problems have been going on for a couple of decades at least. Such research has paid off in several instances, as discussed in the body of this book. Investigations continue in Germany, Italy, Russia, Switzerland and France to find plants that fit the bill, whose active constituents can be found, standardized, and used to prepare the next generation of herbal products: Guaranteed Potency Herbs. Guaranteed Potency Herbs are beginning to answer the often-heard complaint about herbal medicine that one is never certain just how much active material is in any given batch. Guaranteed Potency Herbs are guaranteed by the manufacturer to contain at least the advertised amount of active ingredient. One can, therefore, have considerably more confidence in the reliability of such products.

Cautions.

As revolutionary and exciting as it is, The Guaranteed Potency Herbs concept is not without potential problems. The most serious involves pinning down biological activity to the presence of one constituent or a limited group of constituents. Constituents have to be identified, isolated and tested in living organisms, first animals, then humans. Those tasks are not easy. A second, related, problem concerns the possibility of potential toxicity of the active constituent when it is extracted and concentrated. A third, and also related, problem involves the possibility of interactions between the active and non-active constituents which render the active product more or less ineffective and/or toxic.

Another potential problem is the possibility of leaving active material behind that has properties which were not part of any previous research project. Given the current state of labeling regulation in America, which disallows telling the prospective customer what he can expect from an herbal product, it is possible that people could purchase Guaranteed Potency Herbs expecting to enjoy a benefit no longer present.

There are other possible pitfalls: Which herbs will really benefit from extraction and standardization? Which are more effective in a more natural state? Will the herb lose potency if it is prepared in a form that is more bio-available? The terms bio-active and bio-available sometimes get confused. It is not true that, just because a substance is presented in a form that is easy to digest and assimilate, that it will maintain the same activity in the body. A few examples may demonstrate this point. In order for the A-factors (anthraquinones) of cascara sagrada to be active (as laxatives) they must arrive in the large intestine in virtually the same state in which they enter the body. But, if the A-factors are extracted and concentrated, they will be inactivated in the small intestine. Another case involves certain potent compounds, such as germanium, which, to be safe for human consumption must leave the body in the same state in which they enter. To make them more bio-available will not increase their effectiveness, but it could make them highly toxic.

As an example of the danger of missing active constituents, Russians and Germans have, for many years, extracted and concentrated the valepotriates from valerian root, believing all along that these chemicals accounted for the total activity of the plant. Now, research is showing that the sedative properties may not be restricted to, or even dependent upon, the valepotriates at all. Another example: When the ulcer-protecting and curing constituents of licorice root were isolated and extracted, the resulting product was indeed better than the mother plant, but at the cost of dramatically increased chances of side effects. Later, it was found that the stuff left over after the "active" constituents were extracted was practically as effective as the extract, but without side effects!

I recently picked up some marketing information provided by a company at a trade show. The information described their wonderful new ginger root preparation. It was a freeze-dried extract, and was, undoubtedly, a high quality product. However, the literature I was handed included an abstract of my research on ginger root and motion sickness published in *The Lancet*. The implication, of course, was that their product, being a superior preparation from a technological standpoint, would be better at preventing motion sickness than the primitive stuff I used. And it might be; I don't know — but neither do they. That is the point. In discussing the ginger root studies, I always point out that what made that research possible in the first place was the invention of a new method of administration — the capsule. The method of preparation was the key. Change the method of preparation, and you change the properties. Until basic research is done on freeze-dried products (or any other new and exciting methods of preparation), claims for efficacy are unfounded and can be dangerous. A superior processing method does not guarantee a superior medicinal herb.

The above illustrations will hopefully help the reader understand the _real_ importance of Guaranteed Potency Herbs: superior methods of production combined with good basic research on those preparations. There may legitimately be even better methods of preparation, but so what? Until a good deal of basic and clinical research is done on the medicinal properties of such preparations, their worth as medicinal preparations is uncertain. Meanwhile, let us enjoy the benefits to be derived from the products discussed in this book.

American Involvement: Some Concerns.

The above considerations should be highly visible warning signs to the American Herb Industry. Concerns for safety and efficacy should be uppermost in the priorities of those desiring to manufacture Guaranteed Potency Herbs. Entrepreneurship is a positive attribute of our business; but in the attempt to be the first with the most, there exists the danger of sloppy workmanship. Let us remember the goal of our enterprise: the health of the people. Let us make certain of our technology and science before we expose the public to our products. Let us sell nothing before appropriate biochemical, toxicological and efficacy tests have been performed.

Recommendations. In spite of the limitations and difficulties involved in the Guaranteed Potency Herbs concept, the benefits to be derived from that technology completely justify all legitimate research efforts along this line. It is my hope that such research will go forward, not only in Europe, but in America and Asia. A few guidelines to help direct the effort, to avoid waste and to increase the chances for significant results, are presented here.

1. Since the cost of the end product will be substantially higher than the raw material (which goes into regular herbal products), only such herbs should be selected whose potential medicinal benefits warrant the higher cost. This recommendation is meant to prevent the

standardization and marketing of herbs with questionable value. People, trusting in the wisdom of the industry, would no doubt buy such products; but this kind of exploitation would eventually undermine public confidence.

2. Only herbs with well-established efficacy should be used. Until an herb's efficacy can be established, its standardization is highly suspect.

3. Only herbs whose active constituents have been definitely and unequivocally identified should be used. The temptation is to assume one knows what the active constituents are. Experience in the study of medicinal herbs has taught me that experts in medicinal chemistry are often premature in their judgments about what fraction of a plant contains the major activity. I have little confidence in state-of-the-art approaches to ascertaining active constituents of medical botanicals. The Guaranteed Potency concept only works when you know what should be standardized, and therefore guaranteed. It does little good, and may actually be detrimental, to standardize the *wrong* constituent. The growing tendency among herbal 'experts,' to think they *know* what the active constituents of all herbs are, is dangerous indeed. Even now, I am beginning to hear cries of "Let's standardize everything," a plea that, if heeded, would be a mistake of monumental proportions.

4. All potentially important interactions among the candidate herb's constituents should be explored. This is the most difficult kind of research, even for the manufacturers of the currently available Guaranteed Potency Herbs. In the absence of such research, the final product must contain an adequate complement of whole herb materials. Most of the products discussed in this book fall into that category.

5. In spite of what is known about the herb's toxicity, an entirely separate batch of toxicity tests must be carried out on the potential end product. This will be the criterion most commonly violated by American manufacturers over the next few years.

In view of the above discussion, I would say that serious American involvement in the *production* of new Guaranteed Potency Herbs is highly unlikely during the next decade. Our best course of action is to support the already flourishing European industry, by importing and encouraging public application of products already developed. Limited production of Guaranteed Potency Herbs, with highly standardized manufacturing procedures, that are available to U.S. firms, is also feasible. And limited intercontinental joint ventures in the development of new products are also possible. The ginseng product discussed in this book is an example of European technology (high potency extracts) moderated by American wholistic concerns (use of whole herb).

Guaranteed Potency vs. Wholistic.

One legitimate question is, does the use of Guaranteed Potency Herbs remove us one step from a wholistic approach to health? Being committed, myself, to wholistic health care, I have had to scrutinize the Guaranteed Potency Herbs approach very carefully. There are individuals who believe that any processing of herbal materials is a violation of wholistic medicine. But those people should realize that brewing a tea, grinding, drying, and other "home-grown" procedures are all examples of processing. The encapsulated product is one more degree of processing, but as long as whole herb material is used, I think the capsule can safely be classified as wholistic. Extracts, whether alcohol, apple cider vinegar, glycerin, water, freeze-dried, or whatever, belong in the wholistic camp, as long as they are obtained directly from whole herb material and some attempt is made to retain the natural complement of active constituents.

Guaranteed Potency Herbs also begin and end with whole herb material. But in-between, during the extraction process, the levels of certain key ingredients are measured, and increased, if necessary. This procedure, if done unwisely, may result in the creation of an artificial imbalance between the constituents. In order to prevent the alteration of any medicinal value that depends upon relative concentrations of active ingredients, much research is required to determine the nature of any key interactions among the active ingredients. Without that knowledge, the final product will simply be a best guess.

The determination of key interactions is generally obtained by testing various batches of herb material in physiological systems, recording which are most effective, and measuring the relative levels of all known constituents. Once this work has been done, researchers can attempt to alter subsequent batches of herb to match the relative levels of active constituents in the most effective batch. In other words, the Guaranteed Potency Herbs concept recognizes the inherent variability in plant material, and hence the inherent variability in the *effectiveness* of plant material, and attempts to eliminate the variability from the end product. Panax ginseng, for example, is known to vary greatly in Rg1 concentration. Since the Rg1 fraction is critical for efficacy, quality control specialists make certain the Rg1 fraction is present in a concentration of *at least 50%* of that of the Rb1 fraction; research has shown that this ratio is optimal for best effect. Non-guaranteed potency material will have an unkown amount of Rg1, and, unless the particular batch is one of the best, that is, unless all soil, climatic, harvesting, processing and storage conditions are near perfect, the amount of Rg1 is almost certainly going to be minimal.

The key to the Guaranteed Potency Herb concept is careful adherence to all research and processing stipulations required to insure that key ratios are not disturbed, but rather guaranteed, to be present. When those stipulations are followed, the resulting product conforms very well with the wholistic concept, and may be used by wholistic practitioners with greater confidence than raw material.

Guaranteed Potency vs. Isolates.

Isolates are single constituents that have been extracted (isolated) from the parent herbal material. They are stripped of all their total context. The rationale behind this procedure is that a body of research exists which shows a certain efficacy for the isolate. The rest of the plant material is unnecessary, and may even get in the way (via dilution or unwanted interactions). It should be obvious that Guaranteed Potency Herbs are not the same as isolates. The isolate is not wholistic medicine.

An example of an isolate currently making the rounds in health food stores is pseudo-ephedrine and its derivatives. Psuedo-ephedrine was orginally obtained from certain *ephedra* species, but is currently made synthetically. Its more potent cousin, ephedrine, is obtained from ma huang (ephedrine is also an isolate). Placing these substances in a base of herbs with purportedly similar properties does not in the least detract from the fact that isolates are being used. Pseudo-ephedrine-based drugs have been available in drug stores and supermarkets for years, and they are very good nasal decongestants, anti-allergy, anti-cold symptom type medicines. So here we have an instance of the herb market copying the drug market, except that herb manufacturers are always careful to put the pseudo-ephedrine in a base of herbs. This marketing concept has even become so refined that the same active constituent (pseudo-ephedrine) is sold by the same company under different trade names, depending upon the make-up of the herbal base in which it is placed. Thus one product is for colds, another for hay fever, and so on, but the active ingredient remains the same.

Does the herbal base make a difference? There is currently no research to indicate whether it does or doesn't. *Caveat emptor*.

So far as I am aware, no herb company is currently producing a clone of another well-known cold remedy, one that depends on the presence of another group of isolates, the belladonna alkaloids — atropine, scopolamine and hyosyamine — but I expect that situation will change in the near future.

Herbal isolates have been used as anti-cancer remedies for decades. Most of these are controlled substances, such as the periwinkle alkaloids, vincristine, vinblastine, etc. Licorice root isolate, glycyrrhetinic acid (GA), known medically as cromolyn sodium, has been a popular ulcer treatment in Europe for decades. Periwinkle isolates and GA possess several side-effects.

So far, my treatment of isolates may have seemed harsh. In actuality, there may be a place for them in wholistic medicine, but those discussed above do not fit my concept of safe, preventative, anabolic medicine. And they certainly bear little similarity to Guaranteed Potency Herbs.

However, as with all general rules, there are exceptions. For example, deglycyrrhizinated licorice (DGL), another licorice root isolate, is currently being marketed in United States health food stores as an ulcer treatment. It is better than GA because it lacks side effects (but if you put the two together you have whole licorice root—the reasons for not promoting the whole herb are not clear). Certain antibiotic principles could be extracted from plants and used by themselves or combined with other herbs to produce very effective antibiotic compounds. I can imagine a very good treatment for the stubborn giardia micro-organism being produced by combining very pure concentrates of certain goldenseal and *berberis* alkaloids. And I expect one day to see a very effective anti-insomnia product that depends exclusively on concentrated isolates from hops, passion flower and skullcap. Bromelain, a group of enzymes isolated from the pineapple, is already available, because much research has demonstrated that it can be effective, and, more importantly, delineate the conditions under which it is both useful and effective. Would I call these examples wholistic? No, but I would include them under the wholistic umbrella, as exceptions that prove the rule. I wouldn't recommend them to the exclusion of wholistic products, nor would I recommend their isolated use. But within a fabric built from whole herbs, they could be extremely valuable. There are, then, certain herbal components that could be used much like vitamin and mineral supplements are used within wholistic medicine—not as primary therapeutic agents, but as adjuncts.

Flavonoids may currently be the most beneficial class of isolates available. Scientists have known for some time that much of the medicinal activity of plants can be attributed to the presence of flavonoids (reviewed elsewhere in this book). Quercetin, catechin, rutin and khellin are examples of flavonoids that could find widespread use in the herb industry over the next few years. They exhibit many of the most beneficial physiological effects on the blood, heart, immune system and liver, and are totally non-toxic. Their safety and activity often depends on sensitive interactions with other plant constituents, and for this reason they should not be used as single ingredients or even as the primary ingredient in herbal products. But they could very well be used to boost the flavonoid activity of a combination of flavonoid-containing whole herbs, especially since flavonoids are hard to digest and assimilate.

Conclusion.

Part One of this book is mainly a presentation of the research that has been done on some of the most important Guaranteed Potency Herbs. In the following chapters you will come to understand and appreciate the tremendous amount of work that has gone into making these herbs available in such a form, and you will hopefully get an idea about how they could be of use to you. I do not discuss all available Guaranteed Potency Herbs in this book. Depending upon how well this material is received, there may eventually be a second volume written. If so, it will include some of the glaring omissions from this book, such as *coleus forskohlii* (forskolin), *eleutherococcus senticosis* (siberian ginseng), hawthorn, valerian root, horsetail, etc.

Bilberry
(vacinium myrtillus)

For Veins, Eyes, and Nerves

Guaranteed Potency Constituents.

The anthocyanosides (cyanidine, malvidine, delphynidine, petunidine and peonidiene, among others). *Whole* bilberry fruit extract, in which the level of anthocyanosides has been standardized, is preferable to *isolated* anthocyanosides. The standardized level of active principle should be no less than 15%. Compared to traditional dry bilberry extract, with a maximum anthocyanidene content of 1-2 percent, the concentrate is appreciably more cost effective. This highly concentrated extract (with an extract/fresh fruit ratio of more than 1:100) allows precise manipulation of therapeutic dosages.

Only *vacinium myrtillus* should be used. The North American blueberry (*vacinium myrtilloides*), for example, is unsuitable for standardized medicinal preparation or use.

Industrial research has developed a product that has dramatically reduced experimental error and variability in results. The active constituents of the bilberry, the anthocyanosides, are extremely sensitive to the presence of water, to ascorbic acid, to pH, to the presence of sugar and to polyvalent metallic ions. All of these "contaminants" will reduce the effectiveness of the product. An important production problem has involved the actual concentration of active materials in the extract. The determination of the most effective method of extraction took a great deal of research all by itself. Additional problems included the usual difficulties in the standardization of cultivating and harvesting procedures. And due to the sensitivity of the anthocyanosides to moisture, the storage of both raw and processed product requires the implementation of special low-humidity environments. Only the best manufacturing firms have been able to overcome all of these inherent difficulties. Although early bilberry preparations were observably effective, modern bilberry products are able to exert remarkably reliable and significant effects on the vascular system of the body.

History.

Bilberry fruit has been a popular source of fresh jam for hundreds of years. This berry is native to northern Europe and Asia. The nearest American counterparts are the huckleberry and blueberry. However, only bilberry should be used for standardized medical preparations. Other varieties are unsuitable. Both the leaves and berries of the bilberry bush have been used medicinally, but it is the berry in particular that has yielded the most promising therapeutic data.

One of the most interesting folk/clinical uses for bilberry fruit occurred during World War II, when RAF pilots swore that eating bilberry jam prior to night missions significantly improved night vision (dark adaptation and visual acuity). Such reports stimulated considerable research interest in bilberry in Europe and in South America. Over the course of several years, studies were published that implicated bilberry fruit extract in the effective treatment of a variety of visual problems, including night blindness (nyctalopia), visual fatigue from prolonged reading and working in dim light, severe nearsightedness (myopia) and various vascular disturbances of the retina.

Clinical research on bilberry was being carried out simultaneously with basic research, and actually preceded it. This highly unusual order of experimental investigation was possible because bilberry fruit had been considered a food substance of the purest kind for hundreds of years, even by the establishment. One can see the difference between "feeding" somebody an extract of jam and administering an extract of milk thistle.

Method of Action.

Animal and laboratory studies have revealed much about how bilberry extract works. On the most basic level it increases the resistance of blood capillaries and reduces their permeability. On a more interesting level bilberry affects some major physiological processes. One of the most important of these is the visual apparatus. As we will see, by accelerating the regeneration of retinal purple, bilberry anthocyanosides markedly affects the course of several visual disorders.

The current theory of vision holds that the generation of neural impulses from the retina to the brain depends upon the presence of visual purple (rhodopsin) in the rods (similar mechanisms operate in the cones). Rhodopsin is a simple compound of a protein molecule called opsin and vitamin A. Since the body cannot produce vitamin A, the amount and quality of rhodopsin depends upon the dietary intake of this vitamin. When a molecule of opsin combines with a normally straight molecule of vitamin A the resulting molecule of rhodopsin has a bent shape; the process is much like bending a piece of spring steel. Like a cocked trigger, the rhodopsin is ready to respond to the stimulus of light. When a single photon of light strikes a rod the opsin is forcibly separated from the vitamin A molecule, which snaps back to its straight form thereby releasing enough energy to produce an electrical discharge in an adjoining neuron. As strange as it sounds, the entire process of vision and visual information processing begins with this simple reaction.

Repeated firing of a rod gradually depletes the store of rhodopsin and visual fatigue sets in. In bright light rhodopsin is used up faster than it can regenerate. As the day wanes and darkness comes on, stores of rhodopsin build, the rods regenerate and prepare themselves for the difficult task of night vision. Obviously, the more saturated with rhodopsin rods become the better they are at adapting to the dark.

The process is a marvel and it depends totally on diet. Though the mechanism was not discovered until this century, man has been aware of the connection between diet and sight for more than 4000 years. And without knowing anything about vitamin A, doctors have been recommending foods high in this vitamin for visual problems throughout the ages. Raw liver of donkey, cod liver oil and carrots are just a few of the items known to affect vision. As mentioned above, in the second world war, bilberry acquired a similar reputation.

In laboratory settings, researchers found that the anthocyanosides (pigmentary substances, as is rhodopsin) when administered intravenously to rabbits dramatically sped up the regeneration of rhodopsin and produced remarkably fast dark adaptation.[1] Other studies followed, some utilizing whole extract, others investigating isolated constituents; different animals were used, sometimes isolated visual tissue was examined. In all cases the considerable impact on visual purple was the same.[2-5]

A series of trials uncovered yet another mechanism of action. It appears that bilberry anthocyanosides favorably affect the operation of crucial enzymes in the retinal cellular metabolism and function, such as glucose-6-phosphatase and phosphoglucomutase.[6-7]

While some investigators were looking at the effects of bilberry on adaptation mechanisms, another group of scientists were observing interesting effects on blood capillary stability. Several of these studies utilized the Ambrose and De Eds technique which involves injecting a dyeing agent (normally blue) into a vein and rubbing the bare skin with chloroform. This produces a local irritation and subsequent spreading of the dye into tissues outside of the vein and capillaries.

The rapidity with which the skin turns blue is a measure of the permeability (or leakiness) of the vessels. Bioflavonoids, which decrease the permeability of blood vessels, are known collectively as vitamin P. In one test comparing bilberry anthocyanosides against the best known vitamin P factors, bilberry demonstrated greater intensity and duration of action than any of the others.[8] In another experiment, bilberry extract was compared to vitamin P in their respective effects on rhodopsin. Again, the bilberry was observed to be more effective.[9]

In tests using a number of different species of animals, bilberry anthocyanosides significantly protected vessel walls against the application of vacuum suction, a technique that eventually leads to the total failure of surface vessels.[10] Likewise, in another measure of capillary protection — the inhibition of experimentally induced edema — bilberry has been shown to be very effective.[11]

Highly technical experiments in animals and isolated tissues have demonstrated the ability of bilberry anthocyanosides to protect the blood-brain barrier through a process similar to that exhibited by centella (see chapter on Centella).[12] Further research is needed to explore the implications of these findings.

In other pre-clinical trials bilberry anthocyanosides have been shown to possess the following kinds of activity:

* protection of the heart against the stress of prolonged exposure to swimming as measured by activation of the crucial enzyme lactic dehydrogenase as well as other cardiac enzymes.[13] Other cardio-protective actions of bilberry have been reported. [14]

* possession of good anti-inflammatory activity.[15]

* inhibition of cholesterol-induced atherosclerosis.[16]

* modest inhibition of serum platelet aggregation, thus possessing some anti-thrombotic potential.[17-18]

Therapeutic Research.

Ophthalmology

Inspired by reports coming out of the war, post-World War II physicians began using bilberry fruit extract to treat some specific and rather esoteric ophthalmic conditions such as night blindness,[19] severe myopia,[20] retinal disturbances of various kinds and chronic visual fatigue.[21] The results of these clinical trials were very promising even though there were some problems with standardization of product which led to wide variations in the outcome of therapy.

Doctors throughout Europe and South America began to use crude bilberry extracts and isolated anthocyanosides to treat a wide range of common vision problems. People treated were normally those whose jobs made heavy demands on the visual apparatus. These included airline pilots,[22] air-traffic controllers,[23] car and truck drivers,[24] students, computer terminal operators, navigators,[25] watch makers (and similar professions) and sportsmen of various kinds. Again the results were promising, in that positive results were frequently observed, and again they were plagued by considerable variability in outcome due to lack of controls in subject selection, evaluation techniques, simultaneous administration of other medications, and so forth, as well as the lack of extract standardization.[26] Thus, although it definitely appeared that the extract was working, it was impossible to predict just how well, under what conditions, and for which subjects it would work. What's worse, it was difficult to tell which extraction process would yield the most effective product.

The first *published* clinical experiment was a simple attempt to demonstrate dark adaptation and improvements in visual acuity under controlled conditions in normal human adults. It was one thing to base clinical practice on anecdotal reports from pilots and truck drivers, yet it was quite another to subject such anecdotal evidence to the scrutiny of experimental control. But the results of that study, carried out in 1964 by a team of French scientists, confirmed the anecdotes: dark adaptation, following prolonged exposure to bright light, was significantly accelerated, and some improvement in visual acuity in dim light was observed in experimental subjects.[27] The most obvious effects were observed during the first four hours following ingestion of a single dose of the crude bilberry extract, and almost all effects had worn off after 24 hours.

Similar results were obtained in other early studies. Again, normal healthy subjects were used, and similar positive effects on retinal sensitivity to light were observed.[28-29] We are talking, therefore, about a quick acting substance with practically no residual or long-term habituating action on the body.

It is always a positive feature of medicinal substances if they wear off quickly — this avoids the necessity of carrying out expensive, time-consuming studies on the effects of substance accumulation in about 100 different tissues and organs of the body, and on potential habituating problems.

Results in patients with pigmentary retinitis were similar to those observed in healthy subjects: enlargement of the range of vision as well as a more responsive adaptation to darkness.[30-36] It was the opinion of many investigators that such results in diseased patients were truly remarkable phenomena.

In other studies, bilberry has been effective in aiding hemeralopia (day blindness — the opposite of nyctalopia). In this condition, night vision is only slightly affected, but day vision is greatly impaired, often to the point of total blindness. By the second day of treatment with bilberry, an improvement in retinal luminous sensitivity is observed in many of the patients. Significant improvement remains constant throughout the following three months of treatment, and then gradually diminishes during a subsequent period during which the product is withdrawn. If the treatment is reinstated, improved visual adaptation and acuity are once again observed. No side-effects of any kind are experienced.[37] Such results have been observed more than once.[38]

During the course of research on bilberry's role in improving visual acuity, it became apparent that bilberry anthocyanosides were most effective on those tissues that are sensitive to disturbances in the capillary blood system. The effect of bilberry on vision was not due to a high content of vitamin A, but to a complex network of supportive actions that strengthened capillary integrity and promoted a healthy interplay of important enzymes.

Vascular disorders

As researchers gradually became aware of the true mechanism of action of bilberry anthocyanoside, they became more and more curious about how this substance would affect the course of other disorders involving faulty vascularity. A series of experiments and detailed studies followed.

In one study, patients with blood purpuras, anti-coagulating problems, varicose veins, and various central nervous system circulation problems were successfully treated with bilberry extract.[39]

On another occasion, as part of a doctoral dissertation, bilberry anthocyanosides (then still a very new product) were used to treat 124 cases of various arterial and venous problems and 10 cases of capillary fragility. The results were generally very satisfactory.[40]

An in-depth investigation of the effects of bilberry on hyperpermeability of the capillaries found that treatment restored ionic balance to vessel walls, and eliminated leaks that allowed plasmatic proteins to distribute dangerously on both sides of the membranes.[41] In other studies good results were obtained in conditions ranging from phlebitis to hypertension as long as they involved breakdown of capillary walls (hyperpermeability or fragility).[42-45] Even fragility associated with advanced diabetes is susceptible to bilberry. Several referenced studies report a synergistic action between bilberry anthocyanosides and beta-carotene.

Another line of research demonstrated that bilberry anthocyanosides can have a beneficial effect in persons suffering from the rupture and breakdown of increasingly fragile capillaries in the glomerulus (filtering unit) of the kidneys. The fragility and collapse of these tiny capillaries may result from numerous conditions, including infection, traumatic injury, cancer and various vascular diseases. The major clinical sign is blood in the urine (hematuria), and this sign can be used as the dependent variable for experimental investigation. Many patients exhibiting hematuria experience a significant improvement while using bilberry. Others do not improve. Researchers believe the chances for improvement are related to the seriousness and stage of the underlying disease. The more serious the disease and the more advanced the stage, the less likely it is that bilberry extract will have an observable effect.[46]

Pregnant women suffering from varices and various blood disorders have been treated with anthocyanosides. A combination of bilberry anthocyanosides and vitamin E has proved very effective and seems to be well tolerated; no side effects occur in either mother or infant.[47]

The findings of additional clinical investigations are reported below:

* stimulation of peripheral circulation.[48]

* therapeutic benefits on disorders of the vessels in the conjunctiva of diabetic and pre-diabetic patients with tendencies toward glaucoma.[49]

* anti-spasmodic and central nervous system sedative action.[50]

* inhibition of platelet aggregation, implicated in the prevention of thromboses.[51]

* management of retinal hemorrhage during prolonged anti-coagulant therapy.[52]

All successful applications of bilberry anthocyanosides involve an underlying arterial and/or venous substrate, associated with capillary fragility and/or hyperpermeability, that is corrected by the bilberry extract.

Therapeutic action.

Vision disorders

We have seen that the active constituents of bilberry have been isolated and experimentally verified in clinical trials. In many clinical trials, standardized bilberry extracts, whether administered to healthy human volunteers or to diseased patients, significantly improve night-time visual acuity. They produce quick adjustments to darkness and demonstrably accelerate adjustment to darkness following exposure to a flash of bright light.

The implications for dark adaptation and night time visual acuity are far-reaching. Possible applications are limited only by the imagination. Persons suffering from eye strain of almost any kind will benefit from the use of Guaranteed Potency bilberry extract: students, truck drivers, pilots, those who must stare at computer monitors for extended periods of time, those who constantly work in very dim light or very bright light, and so on.

Additionally, many specific diseases of the visual apparatus may be effectively treated, particularly vascular retinal disturbances, cataracts, diabetic-induced glaucoma, and myopia. Bilberry is one of just a very few compounds known to produce positive effects in the course of macular degeneration.

Vascular disorders

The implications of research on blood vessel or capillary fragility and permeability are not always as clear cut. Several avenues for effective use appear to be open for personal experimentation. First of all, bilberry extract should be an effective treatment for varicose veins and related conditions; it should be a good astringent. Second, it should be an effective anti-coagulant. For example, it has been used in experimental settings in the prevention of thrombosis. Varices of assorted origin should be susceptible to treatment. Third, standardized bilberry extracts should be ideally suited for the careful and precise treatment, and/or relief of, capillary rigidity and permeability-related ailments of many kinds: hypertension, advanced diabetes, arteriosclerosis, purpuras or hemorrhages of the skin, mucous membranes, internal organs and other tissues, brain circulation disorders, kidney hematuria, bleeding gums, etc.

In Europe, standardized bilberry extracts are listed as the primary ingredient in a wide range of proprietary over-the-counter preparations designed specifically for the treatment or relief of the various eye problems discussed in this chapter, disturbances of the central nervous system, varicose veins, and so on. The medicine has become firmly established in European pharmacology.

European products usually contain secondary active ingredients, such as the following: lecithin, citric acid, vitamin E, vitamin C, vitamin A, aspartic acid, vitamin B6, vitamin B12, L-glutamine, and beta-carotene. Bilberry is often found in standardized anti-diabetic preparations, but not often as the primary ingredient.

21

I suspect that we have just scratched the surface of potential benefits to be derived from the use of this herb. Americans, in particular, will be exposed to a whole new area of self-treatment as bilberry extracts become more widely available. Stimulation of research efforts by the entrance of the United States into the market should also be significant. At this point the future indeed "looks bright."

Route of Administration.

By mouth. No other way of administering bilberry extract has ever been seriously proposed. From the earliest experience with just a jam, to the development of modern Guaranteed Potency products, the efficacy of the oral route has always been accepted.

Dosage.

The optimum dosage depends, to some degree, upon the severity of the condition under treatment. However, for most applications, 2-4 25 mg. capsules per day is sufficient. The use of higher doses has never been known to produce adverse side effects, but one must consider the possibility of waste.

Acute or temporary eye strain should require no more than a single application of 2-4 capsules. Individual differences must, of course, be taken into account.

Toxicity.

Anthocyanosides have been shown to be completely non-toxic when administered in the normal manner, i.e., orally. In toxicity tests on mice and rats, no toxicity was observed when the anthocyanosides were administered orally. Intraperitoneal and intravenous administration produce LD50's of very high values, again validating the low toxicity of the product. Since the preferred route of administration is oral, no toxicity should be expected.[53]

References.

1. Alfieri, R & Sole, P. "Influence des anthocyanosides administres par voie parenterale sur l'adaptoelectroretinogramme du lapin." C.R. Soc. Biol., 158, 2338, 1964.
2. Jayle, G.E., Aubry, M. Gavini, M., Braccini, G. "Etude concernant l'action sur al vision nocturne des anthocyanosides extraits de vaccinum myrtillus." Ann. Ocul. (Paris), 198, 556, 1965.
3. Tronche, P., Bastide, P., Komor, J. "Effet des glucosides d'anthocyanes sur al cinetique de regeneration du pourpe retinien chez le lapin." C.R. Soc. Bul., 161, 2473, 1967.

4. Bastide, P., Rouher, F. & Tronche, P. "Rhodosine et anthocyanosides. A propos de quelques faits experimentaux." Bull. Soc. Ophtalm. Fran., **68**, 801, 1968.
5. Plazonnet, B. Bastide, P. & Tronche, P. C.R. Soc. Biol., 162, 1490, 1968.
6. Cluzel, Ch., Bastide, P. & Tronche, P. "Activites phosphoglucomutasique et glucose-6-phosphatasique de la retine et anthocyanosides extraits de vaccinium myrtillus." C.R. Soc. Biol., **163**, 147, 1969.
7. Cluzel, C., Bastide, P., Wegman, R. & Tronche, P. "Activites enzymatiques de la retine et anthocyanosides extraits de vaccinium myrtillus." Biochem. Pharm., 19, 2295, 1970.
8. Demure, G. "Etude experimentale et clinique d'un nouveau facteur vitaminique P: les anthocynosides." These Medecine Clermont, 1964.
9. Pourrat, H., Bastide, P., Dorier, P., Pourrat, A. & Tronche, P. "Preparation et activite therapeutique de quelques glucosides d'anthocyanes." Chim. Therap., **2**, 33, 1967.
10. Bastide, P., Rouher, F. & Tronche, P. "Aspects pharmacologiques de quelques facteurs de protection vasculaire." Bull. Soc. Pharm. Marseille, **17**, 209, 1968.
11. Bonacina, F. & Pacchiano, F. "Attivita complementare degliantocianosidi in un preparato ad azione antiedemigena e capillaro-protettiva." Boll. Chim. Farm., **113**, 540, 1974.
12. Robert, A.M., Godeau, G., Moati, F. & Miskulin, M. "Action of anthocyanosides of vaccinium myrtillus on the permeability of the blood brain barrier.' J. Med., **8**, 321, 1977.
13. Marcollet, M, Bastide, P. & Tronche, P. "Effet angio- protecteur des anthocyanosides de vaccinium myrtillus objective vis-a-vis de la liberation de la lactate deshydrogenase (LDH) et de ses isoenzymers cardiaques chez le rat soumis a une epreuve de nage." C.R. Soc. Biol., **163**, 1786, 1970.
14. Jonadet, m., Meumier, M.T. & Bastide, P. "Anthocyanosides extraits de vitis vinifera, de vaccinium myrtillus et de pinus maritimus. I. Activites inibitrices vis-a-vis de l'elastase in vitro. II. Activites angioprotectrice comparees in vivo." J. Pharm. Belg., **38**, 41, 1983.
15. Bonacina, F., Galliani, G. * Pacciano, F. "Attivita degli antocianosidi nei processi flogistici acuti." Farmaco, ed. pr., **28**, 428, 1973.
16. Kadar, A., Robert, L., Miskulin, M., Tixier, J.M., Breachemier, D. & Robert, A.M. "Influence of anthocyanoside treatment on the cholesterol-induced atherosclerosis in the rabbit." Paroi Arter., **5**, 18l, 1979.
17. Gomez-Serranillos, F.M., Zaragoza, F. & Alvarez, P. "Efectos sobre la agregacion plaquetaria 'in vitro' de los antocianosidos del vaccinium myrtillus L." An. R. Acad. Farm., **49**, 79, 1983.
18. Zaragoza, G.F & De Llano, P.A. "Estudio del efecto antiagregante de los antocianosidos del vaccinum myrtillus en conejos." An. Real. Acad. Farm., in press.
19. Bailliart, J.P. "Tentative d'amelioration de la vision nocturne." Le Medicin de Reserve, **121**, 1969.
20. Ala El Din Barradah, M., Shourkry, I. & Hegazy, M. "Difrarel 100 in the treatment of retinal vascular disorders and high myopia." Bull. Ophth. Soc. Egypt, **60**, 251, 1967.
21. Gil Del Rio, E. "Los antocianosidos del vaccinium myrtillus en oftalmologia." Arch. Soc. Oftal. Hisp.-Amer., **26**, 969, 1966.
22. Chevaleraud, J. & Perdriel, G. "Peut-on ameliorer la vision nocturne des aviateurs." Gaz. Med. de France, **18**, 25 June 1968.
23. Belleoud, L., Leluan, D. & Boyer, Y. "Etude des effets desglucosides d'anthocyanes sur la vision nocturne des controleurs d'approche d'aerodrome." Rev. Med. Aero. Spat., **5**, 45, 1966.
24. Rouher, F. & Sole, P. "Peut-on ameliorer la vision nocturnedes conducteurs automobiles." Ann. Med. Accidents Traffic, 3-4, 1965.
25. Belleoud, L, Leluan, D & Boyer, Y. "Etude des effets des glucosides d'anthocyanes sur al vision nocturne du personnel navigant." Rev. Med. Aero. Spat., **6**, 5, 1967.
26. Alfieri, R., Sole, P. & Rouher, F. "Action et mecanisme des anthocyanosides dans la vision nocturne." Vie Medic., dic. 1969.
27. Jayle, G.E. & Aubert, L. "Action des glucosides d'anthocyanes sur la vision scotopique et mesopique du sujet normal." Therapie, **19**, 171, 1964.
28. Volpi, U. & Bertoni, G. "L'azione del 'pourpranyl' sulfa sinsibilita luminosa retinica

del soggetto normale." Ann. Ottal. Clin. Ocul., **90**, 492, 1964.

29. Mercier, A., Perdriel, G. & Carves, H. "Note concernant l'activite des glucosides d'anthocyanes sure la vision scotopique et l'acuite visuelle mesopique des sujets normaux." Rev. Med. Aero., 13, 57, 1965.

30. Fiorini, G. Bianacci, A. & Graziano, F.M. "Modificazioni perimetriche ed adattometriche dopo ingestione di mirtillina associata a beta-carotene." Ann. Ottalm. Clin. Ocul., **91**, 371, 1965.

31. Mercier, A., *et. al.* "Note concernant l'action des glucosides d'anthocyanes sur l'electroretinogramme humain." J. Bull. Soc. Ophtalm. Fr., **65**, 1049, 1965.

32. Scialdone, D. "L'azione delle antocianine sul senso luminoso." Ann. Ottal. Clin. Ocul., **92**, 43, 1966.

33. Alfieri, R. & Sole, P. "Influence des anthocyanosides administres par voie oroperilinguale sur l'adapto-electroretinogramme (AERG) en lumiere rouge chez l'homme." C.R. Soc. Biol., **160**, 1590, 1966.

34. Magnasco, A. & Zingirian, M. "Influenza degli antocianosidi sulla soglia retinica differenziale mesopica." Ann. Ottal. Clin. Ocul., **92**, 188, 1966.

35. Goria, E. & Peria, A. "Effetto degli antocianosidi sulla soglia visiva assoluta." Ann. Ottalm. Clin. Ocul., **92**, 595, 1966.

36. Urso, G. "Azione degli antocianosidi del vaccinium myrtillus associati a beta-carotene sulla sensibilita luminosa." Ann. Ottal. Clin. Ocul., **93**, 931, 1968.

37. Zavarisse, G. "Sull'effetto del trattamento prolungato con antocianosidi sul senso luminoso." Ann. Ottal. Clin. Ocul., **94**, 209, 1968.

38. Jueneman, G. "Ueber die wirkung der anthozyanoside auf die hemeralopie nach chininintoxikation." Augenheilkunde, **151**, 891, 1968.

39. Terrasse, J. & Moinade, S. "Premiers resultats obtenus avec un nouveau facteur vitaminique P 'Les anthocyanosides' extraits du v. myrtillus." Presse Med., **72**, 397, 1964.

40. Demure, G. *op. cit.*

41. Cuvelier, R., Terrasse, J., Derycke, Ch., Andraud, G. & Aublet-Cuvelier, J.L. "Essai d'appreciation par le test de landis de l'action sur les capillaires d'un complexe anthocianique." Clermont Med., **63**, 61, 1966.

42. Thomas, Ch. & Barisain, P. "L'action des anthocyanosides sur al fagilite des capillaires oculaire dans le diabete et l'hypertension arterielle." Bull. Soc. Ophtalm. Fran., **65**, 212, 1965.

43. Sevin, R. & Cuendet, J.F. "Effets d'une association d'anthocyanosides de myrtille et de beto-carotene sur la resistance capillaire des diabetiques." Opthalmologica, **152**, 109, 1966.

44. Coget, J. & Merlen, J.F. "Etude clinique d'un nouvel agent de protection vasculaire, le Difrarel 20, composé d'anthocyanosides isoles de v. myrtillus." Phlebologie, **2**, 221, 1968.

45. Guermonprez, J.L. & Miltgen M. "Action des anthocyanosides de vaccinium myrtillus sure la resistance capillaire chez l'hypertendu et la diabetique (a propos de 40 observations)." Vie Med., avril 1972/73.

46. Romeuf, J.C. "Essai clinique d'un facteur vitaminique P sur les hematuries microscopiques." These-Univ. Clermont-Fd., Faculte Mixte de Medicine et de Pharmacie, 1967.

47. Baudon, J., Bruhat, M., Plane, C. & Hermabessiere, J. "Utilisation d'une association d'angio-protecteur et de vitamine E." Lyon Medit. Medical, **46**, ott. 1969.

48. Terrasse, J., Aubiet-Cuvelier, J.L. & Marcheix, J.C. "Action des anthocyanosides sur la circulation peripherique et le test de Landis." Vie Medicale, Dic., 1969.

49. Romani, J.D. "Action des anthocyanosides sur l'angiopathie conjonctivale au cours du diabete et du prediabete." Vie Medicale, Dic., 1969.

50. Canivet, J. & Passa, Ph. "Interet therapeutique d'une association d'anthocyanosides, d'antispasmodiques et de neuro-sedatif central." G.M. de France, **78**, 682, 1971.

51. Rasmussen, Ch. "Anthocyanosides. Adhesivite plaquettaire et prevention des thromboses." Therapeutique, **48**, 399, 1972.

52. Neumann, L. "Erfahrungen mit anthocyanosid-behandlung von netzhautblutungen unter antikoagulantien-dauertherapia." Augenheilkunde, **163**, 96, 1973.

53. Pourrat H., et. al., 1967, *op. cit.*

Butcher's Broom
(ruscus aculeatus)

For Varicose Veins, Hemorrhoids and Other Vein Disorders

Guaranteed Potency Constituents.

Ruscogenins. These saponins should be present in a 10% concentration. Whole butcher's broom should be used, since isolated ruscogenins may not possess the same activity or lack of toxicity as whole plant materials. Butcher's broom products that are not carefully manufactured are often found to be seriously lacking in ruscogenin content. Like all saponins, the ruscogenins are steroidal in structure. Ruscogenin is the aglycone of ruscin. Neo-ruscogenin, another steroidal saponin, is also biologically active, and its presence in the guaranteed potency herb preparation is counted with ruscogenin. This is done, even though the two aglycones occur in variable amounts of each, depending on the region where the butcher's broom rhizomes were gathered, because the two chemicals are almost identical, both in chemistry and in activity. The aglycones are more similar to each other than are isomers (which are identical except for rotation); neo-ruscogenin simply has one more double bond than ruscogenin.

History.

The folklore history of butcher's broom dates back to the time of Greek civilization. Laxative and diuretic uses for the *whole* plant were described by Dioscorides. The plant grew abundantly in the Mediterranean region, from the Azores to Iran, and was, therefore, widely used by the people of these areas. European herbalists recommended butcher's broom for various ailments, including the mending of broken bones, but despite such recommendations, butcher's broom never became a very popular herb.

It wasn't until the middle of this century that a truly promising use for the plant was found. And then it was not the herb, but the rhizomes (underground stems) of the plant, that contained the active principles. The ruscogenins were discovered during the routine search for new sapogenins suitable for use as raw materials in the preparation of steroids. French scientists were the first to reveal that butcher's broom extract possessed vasoconstriction (blood vessel narrowing) and anti-inflammatory properties. Since that time, the extract has become very popular in European medicine as a treatment for venous circulatory disorders (especially for women complaining of a heavy sensation in the legs), as well as hemorrhoidal ailments.

In the United States, butcher's broom remedies have been available for some time. The advertising claims associated with some of these products have claimed that the herb is "rare." This is not true. What is rare is a product that contains standardized, guaranteed potency butcher's broom, of whose reliability one can be assured.

Method of Action.

Reports from the early '50's showed that simple alcohol extracts of whole butcher's broom rhizomes were very effective in constricting peripheral blood vessels.[1-4] Concomitant toxicological screenings suggested that the herb was extremely safe to use, much more than other preparations being used to treat hemorrhoids. Based on the low toxicity findings, several pharmaceutical houses quickly prepared creams, salves and ointments for testing as external applications to hemorrhoids in human patients. The results (discussed below) were highly significant. Clinical trials with external preparations have been supported down through the years by continued pharmacological investigation of the vasoconstrictive effects.[5-9] Besides the simple vasoconstrictor action, butcher's broom tones up a sluggish venous system and reduces capillary fragility. An enzymatic effect reduces pain and swelling. Insufficient circulation to the extremities is reversed. This pertains also to circulation problems involving the retina.

It wasn't until the mid '60's and later, that the anti-inflammatory property of butcher's broom was established.[10-12] In carrageenin and beer yeast-induced edema studies, butcher's broom demonstrated good anti-inflammatory effects compared to several standard anti--inflammatory drugs. It was somewhat surprising that it took ten years to clearly demonstrate the anti-inflammatory effect, since vaso-dilation was part of the inflammatory process, and butcher's broom had already been shown to constrict blood vessels. At any rate, since a great many vascular problems were associated with inflammation, this finding suggested even more uses for butcher's broom.

Perhaps the most extensive pharmacological study was conducted in Europe in 1972.[13] This study not only compared the anti-inflammatory effect of butcher's broom with several additional agents, it reported good efficacy of butcher's broom in other aspects. For example, butcher's broom reduced the permeability of diseased capillaries in the rabbit, and thereby stabilized the flow of nutrients, toxins and other particulate matter across venous membranes. But it did not have this effect on capillaries in rats. The reasons for this species difference are not clear. No changes in blood pressure were noted, nor was any toxic activity seen in heart muscle preparations. The hemolytic (rupture of red blood cells with release of hemoglobin into the plasma) action of butcher's broom, unlike that of many anti-inflammatory agents, proved negligible, even when doses were adjusted for equal anti-inflammatory action.

Other variables that were measured during long periods of butcher's broom ingestion included body weight, blood sugar levels, hepatic function, diuresis, electrolyte secretion, and morphological/anatomical appearance of cells, blood and organs. No significant changes were seen in any of these variables, indicating a singular lack of toxicity in butcher's broom. Butcher's broom thus emerges from the basic research literature as a potent, yet totally safe, therapeutic agent.

Therapeutic Research.

Clinical research with the ruscogenins has not been plentiful outside Europe, but on the continent the preparation is recognized for its usefulness in treating hemorrhoids and venous problems involving inflammation, such as are discussed in the section following this one. Widespread European use has resulted in the proliferation of loosely controlled clinical trials, most of which substantiate the medical claims.

Much of the pre-clinical work has involved simultaneous administration to human patients. Since hemorrhoids and varicose veins are not considered life threatening, research standards are much less strict. Human trials are permissible so long as no signs of toxicity are observed.

Hemorrhoids

So far most research on butcher's broom has been done on hemorrhoids and related conditions. Without attempting a lengthy review of that rather mundane and repetitious research here, we can summarize by stating that the vast majority of results were positive. The signs and symptoms of both external and internal hemorrhoids, including bleeding, itching, soreness, and swelling, have been successfully treated with repeated application of butcher's broom, over several days or weeks. Inflammatory states of the ano-rectal mucosa were quickly reduced in size (and pain), and the return of a healthy appearance was achieved within a short time.[14-18]

Circulation disorders

Circulation disorders of the legs have also been the subject of considerable research activity. Dramatic improvement in both subjective and objective measures is observed within days. The ubiquitous "heaviness in the legs" symptom, commonly reported by mothers and working women, responds to treatment, in most studies, within days to a few weeks. More resistant to permanent alteration, but still capable of cure, are varicose veins, varicose ulcers, and surface veins.[19-20] Phlebitis, resulting from insufficient circulation, and associated complications ranging from edema to varices, have all yielded to treatment with butcher's broom. In ophthalmological trials, such conditions as diabetic retinopathy (including microaneurysms and punctate exudates) and retinal hemorrhaging have been successfully treated with butcher's broom.

Post-operative recovery

In hospital settings, butcher's broom has been used to accelerate post-operative recovery, especially where there was prolonged and heavy bleeding, or when anti-coagulant therapy was being administered, or in patients suffering from phlebitis.[21-22] Finally, research has shown that chilblains (a common vasomotor disorder of the extremities) can be successfully treated with butcher's broom. Chilblains are usually the result of sensitivity to cold, brought on by circulatory disturbances (not to be confused with frostbite). The toning effect of butcher's broom on the peripheral capillaries could be responsible for its therapeutic effect on chilblains. The herb would increase the flow of blood through affected tissues. Chilblains arising from other causes are not susceptible to treatment with butcher's broom.

Therapeutic Action.

The most immediate and obvious use for butcher's broom is in the treatment of hemorrhoids and related conditions. We can look to the Europeans for examples.

In Europe, butcher's broom, as a tablet, salve or suppository, is recommended and used by the medical profession for the treatment of internal and external hemorrhoids (internally and externally), hemorrhoidal bleeding, inflamed and bleeding hemorrhoids, inflammation and bleeding of the vicinity around the rectum, before and after the surgical removal of hemorrhoidal knots, proctitis, pruritus ani (rectal itching) and anal fissures. It works by rapidly decreasing inflammation and pain and by strengthening the capillaries that feed this area. Butcher's broom appears to be one of the best treatments for hemorrhoids currently available, and that includes all known drugs and herbal preparations.

For applications other than hemorrhoids, butcher's broom is usually combined with other Guaranteed Potency herbs with similar properties such as centella and bilberry. These preparations are recommended in the treatment of postthrombotic syndrome, venous circulatory disturbances such as chilblains, peripheral circulatory edema, varicophlebitis, pregnancy- related varicose veins (e.g., milk leg), varicose ulcers, and post- operative venous disorders, and other disorders of the peripheral hemodynamic. Thousands of European women take daily advantage of the ability of butcher's broom to augment the tone and elasticity of capillary walls, by using the herb in the treatment of "heaviness in the legs;" thousands of others use it to help reduce edema experienced after standing at work all day; and an equal number of people apply it in the attempt to get rid of surface veins. How much success is experienced by the latter is unknown, but widespread application speaks for itself.

Another use for butcher's broom, one that is becoming more common, is the treatment of retinal hemorrhages and diabetic retinopathy.

Gynecological applications of butcher's broom are also becoming more common. Women report that it helps alleviate menstrual problems, troubles associated with the use of estrogens, and pregnancy-related cramps.

In summary, butcher's broom may be applied as follows:

Proctology: Hemorrhoids, external and internal, proctitis, pruritus ani (rectal itching) and anal fissures.

Phlebology: Varicose veins, varices, chilblains, "heavy" legs, surface veins, postthrombotic syndrome, other venous circulatory disturbances, peripheral circulatory edema (swelling), varicophlebitis, (e.g., milk legs), varicose ulcers, and post-operative venous disorders, and other disorders of the peripheral hemodynamic.

Ophthalmol: Diabetic retinopathy, retinal hemorrhages.

Gynecology: Menstrual problems, troubles with estrogens, cramps of pregnancy, varicose veins of pregnancy.

Route of Administration.

There are three normal ways to use butcher's broom. The most common is the capsule; this is the traditional preparation for prevention and treatment of venous circulation problems. Encapsulated butcher's broom may also be taken internally as an adjunct in the treatment of hemorrhoids.

However, normal proprietary preparations for hemorrhoid treatment are the ointment and suppository. Home remedy equivalents for those two preparations are available: poultice, compress, salve, ointment, suppository, bolus, herbal tea enema. By separating the capsule, you can use the material contained therein to produce preparations that can be used for external application to the rectal area, and for rectally administered "internal" application. A few examples are presented below.

A poultice is prepared by combining the herb powder with a small amount of hot water to form a thick, moist paste. This is applied directly to the inflamed and swollen tissues.

A simple ointment is obtained by mixing one part powdered herb with four parts melted lard (other fats can be used, but they must be hard at room temperature). A bit of gum benzoin may be added to the ointment to preserve it. Another simple ointment is prepared by mixing the powder (2-3 capsules) in vaseline (teaspoon). The two should be gently simmered together for 5-10 minutes. More complicated ointments can be made; consult your favorite herbal for directions. And experiment.

A bolus, or suppository, of butcher's broom is prepared by mixing the powder into cocoa butter until it forms a thick, doughy mass. Refrigerate overnight and allow to warm up to room temperature the next day. Next, roll it into pieces of rope that are about 1/2 to 1 inch thick and 1 inch long. You insert these pieces directly into the rectum, preferably at night; the herbs are activated as the cocoa butter melts. Wear something, or wrap yourself in something, that will protect bedding from stains. More complicated suppositories are possible; again review the recommendations of your favorite herbalist.

Dosage.

A daily dose of 100 mg., taken internally, is recommended by most manufacturers, and is generally supported by the research literature. Much more than that has been administered for extended periods, without side effects, and has usually resulted in more rapid healing.

Applied externally, as poultice, ointment, bolus or suppository, as much can be applied as desired.

Toxicity.

Side effects, outside of occasional nausea or gastritis, are not known to have occurred using therapeutic doses. Studies on toxicity have shown a remarkable lack of such effects, even at high doses.[23]

References.

1. Caujolle, F., Stanilas, W., Roux, G. & Labrot, P. "Recherches pharmacologiques sur l'intrait de ruscus aculeatus L." 69e Congres Assoc. Fr. Avanc. Sci., Toulose, 1950.
2. Caujolle, F. Meriel, P. & Stanilas, E. "Sur la valeur du fragon en medication antihemorroidaire." Therapie, 7, 428, 1952.
3. Caujolle, F. Meriel, P. & Stanilas, E. "Sur les proprietes pharmacologiques de ruscus aculeatus L." Ann. Pharm. Franc., 11, 109, 1953.
4. Moscarella, C. "Contribution a l'etude pharmacologique du ruscus aculeatus L. (fragon epineux)." These de Pharmacie, Toulouse, 1953.
5. Capra, C. "Studio farmacologico e tossicologico di componenti del ruscus aculeatus L." Fitoterapia, 43, 99, 1972.
6. Tarayre, J.P. & Lauressergues, H. "Etude de quelques proprietes pharmacologiques d'une association vasculotrope." Ann. Pharm. Franc., 34, 375, 1976.
7. Tarayre, J.P. & Lauressergues, H. "Action anti-oedemateuse d'une association enzymes proteolytiques, flavonoides, heterosides de ruscus aculeatus et acide ascorbique." Ann. Pharm. Franc., 37, 191, 1979.
8. Marcelon, G., Verbeuren, T.J., Lauressergues, H. & Vanhoutte, P.M. "Effect of ruscus aculeatus on isolated canine cutaneous veins." Pharmacology, 14, 103, 1983.
9. Rubanyi, G., Marcelon, G. & Vanhoutte, P.M. "Effect of temperature on the responsiveness of cutaneous veins to the extract of ruscus aculeatus." Gen. Pharmac., in press.
10. Chevillard, L, Ranson, M. & Senault, B. "Activite anti-iflammatoire d'extraits de fragon epineux (ruscus aculeatus L.)." Med. Pharmacol. Exp., 12, 109-114, 1964.
11. Cahn, J., Herold, M. & Sanault, B. "Antiphlogistic and anti-inflammatory activity of F 191." Int. Symp. Non Steroidal Anti-inflammatory Drugs. Milano, 1964.
12. & 13. Capra, C. op. cit., 1972.
14. Lemozy, J., Suduca, P., Garrigues, J.M., & Saint-Pierre, A. "Interet du proctolog dans le traitment des hemorroides et des fissures anales." Mediterranee Med., 92, 87, 1976.
15. Chabanon, R. "Experimentation du proctolog dans les hemorroides et les fissures anales." Gaz. Med. de France, 83, 3013, 1976.
16. Pris, J. "Proctolog: utilisation dans un service d'hematologie." Gaz. Med. France, 84, 2423, 1977.
17. Caujolle, F., et. al., op. cit., 1952.
18. Moscarella, C., op. cit., i1953.
19. Cohen, J. "Fraitement par le ruscus des incidences veineuses de la contraception orale." Vie Medicale, X, 1305, 1977.
20. Sterboul, Krawiecki, "Etude clinique d'un vasomoteur veineux. Extrait de fragon epineux." Gaz. Hop. Civils et Militaires, 134, 375, 1962.
21. Verne, J.M., de Montrichard, C. Chevillard, L. & Ranson, M., Ann. de Chirurgie, 14, 1221-51, 1960.
22. & 23 Capra, C., op. cit., 1972.

Centella
(centella asiatica)

For Connective Tissues, Veins, Skin

Guaranteed Potency Constituents.

Asiaticosides and other triterpenes, considered as a group. Highly concentrated extracts of certain *isolated* constituents are available, but the current body of experimental data suggests the possibility of significant interactions among the various triterpenes. For this reason, the *whole* herb, with a guaranteed amount of triterpenes, should be used; this is highly preferable to isolated extracts. Research on several centella species also suggests that a *combination of total triterpenes* is most effective.[1] As to the concentration of triterpenes, one should expect about 10%; this level is currently only available in the Madagascar variety of centella (the particular variety should be specified on labels — if it isn't, it probably isn't Madagascaran). Indian and Ceylonese centella are very low in active constituents.

Centella does not contain caffeine nor any of its analogues.

History.

Centella is native to subtropical and tropical climates. The best varieties are cultivated in Madagascar; India is another important cultivation locale, primarily in the areas around Bombay and Calcutta. Centella leaf is officially recognized in pharmacopeias throughout Asia.

Centella has a remarkable history of use. Asian medicine has relied upon this plant for hundreds of years, for the treatment of skin sores and infections. K. Heyne, in his now classic volumes on the useful plants of Asia, remarked that the plant was equivalent to an entire drug store.[2] It is used extensively in the Ayurvedic system where it is called 'Brahmi' (though this term has apparently also been applied to other plants). Both allopathic and homeopathic medical systems have, at one time or another, used centella to treat problems of the skin, blood and nerves. It is also routinely used as a mild diuretic and a tonic. In the previous century, Indian doctors successfully treated

syphilis.[3] In this century, in India, doctors have been equally successful in treating leprosy with centella.[1] Small amounts are said to stimulate the appetite and aid digestion.

In both Western and Eastern traditions, centella has gained a
solid reputation as a nerve tonic. It is used to increase, in ways currently unknown, the ability to remember and learn.[41] It is also used to help
overcome certain forms of mental illness, especially schizophrenia. For
such purposes, centella is more often combined with other nerve tonics
than used by itself. In addition, there is some evidence that centella
constituents are sedative.[42] It has even found its way into headache
and vertigo remedies.

The antibiotic (bacteriostatic) properties of centella have been
well-documented in experimental trials.[5] In clinical practice, the herb
is used to treat many different kinds of inflammation, infection and
fever. The therapeutic use of centella, in the treatment of skin and
blood disorders, probably depends to some degree on the bacteriostatic
property. In China, centella is said to be a 'cooling' herb, and is used to
reduce fever and detoxify the blood. In actual practice that means
using it for acute infections and inflammations of the skin externally
and internally, as well as drinking a tea to help clear the upper respiratory tract during infection (whooping cough, tightness in chest). This
practice is shared by several Southeast Asian countries. The method of
action for the antibiotic property is fairly well understood.

Finally, we must touch upon the most controversial use of centella: to increase longevity. The first "case history" of such an effect
was that of the ancient Chinese herbalist, LiChing Yun, who purportedly lived for 256 years. Since then, many are the tales coming from
obscure regions of India, Pakistan and Madagascar, of people living
beyond 100 years, while still laboring in the fields. Sri Lankans
purportedly accept centella as a longevity plant on the basis that
elephants eat it — and look how old they get! And it's all attributed to
the use of centella (and other similar-acting plants).

Method of Action.

Research on the method of action of centella began in 1949 with
the isolation of the active asiaticosides by a team of Madagascaran
researchers.[4] These men injected asiaticosides directly into leprosy
nodules, perforated ulcers and lesions on fingers and eyes. The treatment, it was thought, broke down these structures (i.e., dissolved the
waxy covering of the leprosy bacillus so that it became fragile and
vulnerable) leading the way to subsequent healing.

Later, in the '50's, researchers proposed two hypotheses to

account for the effectiveness of centella teas and poultices in the treatment of leprous sores and skin tuberculosis.[6] First, it was possible that the herb's bacteriostatic action (ability to neutralize bacterial activity) accounted for the effect. This was the most logical hypothesis at the time. Thousands of plants throughout the world were known to contain powerful antibiotic substances. In the case of centella, it was necessary to simply assume that its particular triterpenoids were selectively effective against the most destructive bacteria known to man.

It became evident early on, however, that something was wrong with the hypothesis. Test-tube, petri dish, animal and clinical tests clearly indicated that asiaticoside did not act even remotely similar to known antibiotics such as streptomycin.

Meanwhile, another hypothesis was being developed which eventually proved more fruitful. The clue for the development of the second theory was to be found in the observation that rats treated with asiaticoside *healed* much more rapidly than controls, and with a considerably lower mortality rate. The researchers proposed that the asiaticoside was selectively stimulating the "**reticuloendothelial system**," (RES). The RES is a vast network of cells and tissues, found throughout the body, that are concerned with the formation and destruction of blood cells, the storage of fatty materials, the metabolism of iron and pigment, and with inflammation and immune responses. The RES is concentrated in the blood, connective tissue, spleen, liver, lungs, bone marrow and lymph nodes. Some of these cells move freely through the system, responding to "distress calls" from distant points. Many RES cells are *phagocytic*, that is, their primary mission is to ingest and destroy unwanted foreign material. Spleen RES cells can destroy disintegrated or used-up red blood cells, liberating the hemoglobin, which can then be transformed into bile pigments by other RES cells located in the blood cavities of the liver, the connective tissue, and bone marrow. Centella asiaticosides stimulate this system in some interesting ways.[6]

The health and healing of the skin, especially the outer layer, called the epidermis, is fully dependent on the functioning of the RES. During the healing process, especially, certain cells in the epidermis produce a substance known as *keratin*, a protein that is the principle component of skin, nails, hair, even tooth enamel. The process whereby cells produce keratin is known, of course, by as long a term as could be found: "keratinization." One of the ways in which asiaticoside stimulates the RES is by increasing keratinization, the foundation process for building new skin in areas of infection: sores, ulcers, and so forth.[7]

In 1968, it was found that asiaticoside influences skin epidermis by activating the cells of the *stratum germinativum* (the innermost layer of the epidermis); it also stimulates keratinization in ways previously observed. In other words, this research confirmed and extended that of earlier scientists.[8]

Over a period of several years, researchers determined that centella significantly stimulated the synthesis or generation of lipids and proteins important to the health of the skin; it markedly improved the production of hyaluronic acid (the connective "jello" in which cells are suspended) and chondroitinsulfate (a similar substance found in cartilage);[9] it had an express anabolic effect on the metabolism of amino acids.[10] In fact these components were affected even more strongly than keratin production. Significantly, the stimulation of new cell growth was not affected at all. It appears that centella's primary mode of action is on various phases of cellular metabolism within the body's connective tissue, resulting in the development of normal connective tissue, which underlies a correct process of healing. This action differs from that of other healing agents, that stimulate an "artificial" or incorrect healing process by directly increasing the proliferation of new skin. We are talking about a difference that might loosely be called "within versus without." Stimulating the "within" metabolic processes, that are normally responsible for the growth of new tissue in areas of damage, may be viewed as a vastly superior process than stimulating the multiplication of cells from "without."

Asiaticosides from centella may be administered in various ways, the usual being either topically or orally. Following oral administration the asiaticoside remains in the blood for a fairly long time.[11] Three to five per cent may still be in the body 3-5 days later,[12] during which time it is being broken down by enzymatic action in the colon.

Therapeutic Research.

Since about 1979, medicinal preparations containing the triterpenes of centella have been in widespread use (but not in the United States). They are primarily targeted at cellulitis and related conditions involving severe infection and acute inflammation of the skin.

Sclerosis

In one of the earliest trials, scientists administered an extract of centella to subjects every day for three months. They found that tissues, taken from the thigh bone and the deltoid muscle of these subjects, exhibited a significantly reduced tendency to hardening (sclerosis) as a result of inflammation when compared to tissues taken from placebo control subjects.[13] This procedure is recognized by medical researchers as a good one for finding potentially effective anti-sclerotic agents for treatment of arteriosclerosis, and for screening out substances that hold little promise. Passing this trial opened the door for a great variety of clinical trials.

Skin ulcers

Clinically, centella triterpenes are used whenever it is desirable to promote or accelerate the healing of the skin. As far back as 1958, positive research along these lines was being performed.[15] In many studies, all patients with ulcers of the lower limbs were successfully treated. Several of these cases were caused by some kind of alteration in venous circulation. Most had been unsuccessfully treated with other agents. In some cases eczematoid manifestations around the ulcer healed more rapidly than usual. This kind of skin rash is especially prevalent in patients confined to bed for long periods.[16-20]

Clincial trials of this nature usually take place in hospitals and involve patients recovering from surgery or chronic disease. Being confined to hospital beds for extended periods of time produces problems unrelated to the reason the patient went to the hospital in the first place, but which can keep the patient hospitalized longer than necessary or expected. Such problems usually involve more or less severe bed sores and ulcerations, conditions euphemistically known as "traumatic and varicose ulcerative lesions of the limbs." The application of centella triterpenes often results in the rapid shedding of damaged tissues, the intense formation of new epithelial and connective tissues, and a greatly shortened hospital stay.

An example of such research: In 1982, researchers reported a series of trials comprising 27 patients with lesions of various types, such as varicose and arterial ulcers, bedsores, burns and wounds. All cases experienced rapid and definite improvement with complete cleansing of the lesion and formation of healthy new tissue.[20]

Gynecology

During childbirth painful tears, lesions, sores, abrasions, surgical incisions may occur. Troublesome infections are often created by the hospital setting itself — this, in spite of the great care taken by hospital staff to minimize the risk. Day to day care of women who have just delivered requires immediate and effective treatment of infected sores around sutures, both internally and externally. The use of anti-biotics is often counter productive as they can actually lower the natural resistance of the body. It is better to use natural therapy; therefore doctors are always seeking better methods of control. Centella has proved itself worthy of much praise by practicing physicians as well as by basic researchers as a premier gynecological agent.

A great variety of lesions and ulcerative problems associated with pregnancy and delivery have been successfully treated with centella. Cervical lesions of several types, some of up to 50 days duration, were treated in one study. The result was the rapid generation of a uniform, normal-looking mucosa in all cases.[21]

In a series of vigorous trials into its ability to heal small perineal lesions occurring during delivery and obstetric manipulations, centella significantly improve the chances of rapid healing if applied early.[22-23] Administering the extract later always accelerated the healing of tears that failed to heal on their own. In all cases, healing was usually complete in 4 to 6 days, and follow-ups, one or two months later, revealed uniformly good healing.[23] These studies, done in the early 1960's, were unique in that no other agent at that time had been found to act on the healing process itself.

In 1961, centella triterpenes were applied topically in a small number of cases of displacement (ectopia) of the intracervical mucosa. The investigators concluded that the treatment was a good solution to this important problem in cervical pathology.[24]

An extract of centella was used to treat over 50 cases of radiation ulcers in gynecological patients. It resulted not only in the rapid healing and repair of normally slow-healing lesions, but, unlike any other known agent, it also produced a remarkable elasticity and mobility in the scar tissue.[25]

Episiotomy, an incision of the vulva, sometimes performed during the second stage of delivery to avoid later tearing, often results in a very uncomfortable healing process. Mercurochrome and novocaine ointments are traditionally used to lessen pain and chances of infection. Compared to these treatments, extracts of centella yield consistently better results. Almost all women receiving centella reported less pain and more rapid healing than women subjected to standard measures.[26] Doctors report that they like centella so much they apply it as early as possible in the episiotomy healing process.

Ear, nose, throat

Centella triterpenes have been investigated for their effects on the healing process following tonsillectomy and other surgical procedures involving the ear, nose and throat. Normally, repair of the mucosa following tonsillectomy is left to itself. If you heal, fine; if you don't, too bad— eventually you will. But, in comparing the results of 67 patients receiving centella with 67 that did not, it became obvious to the investigating scientists that centella administration resulted in significantly more rapid healing of the tonsillectomy cavities.[27]

One of the main problems involved in radiation surgery of the ear, nose and throat is that the skin, mucosa and blood vessels are extremely slow to heal following the procedure. In many such cases, a normal surgical procedure is followed by some form of radiotherapy. It is during the therapy that healing is inhibited. The use of centella extract in treating several dozen patients, the majority of whom had undergone laryngectomy or pharyngolaryngectomy followed by radiotherapy, yielded extremely encouraging results. Based on clinical observations, investigators have selected the centella extract as the drug of choice to use following such operations.[28,40]

Cellulitis

Many people have experienced cellulitis without realizing what they had. The word is not frequently used, even by doctors, in describing symptoms or disease. More often one hears statements like, "I've got this bad infection." Cellulitis is defined as a diffuse inflammatory process within bodily tissues. It is characterzied by swelling, redness, pain. It is usually the result of infection by streptococci or staphylococci, but other organisms may be involved. Cellulitis may occur in tissues beneath the skin or mucous membranes or around muscle bundles and surrounding organs.

Cellulitis is not to be confused with cellulite, a non-medical term used to refer to the ugly accumulation of subcutaneous fat and water in the hips. It is doubtful that centella would have a direct effect on the latter condition other than that of increasing the tensil strength of the skin and of repairing any underlying damage to connective tissues. It certainly won't have a direct effect on fatty tissues.

One of the most common forms of cellulitis is known as *erysipelas*, a surface inflammation of the skin. Red patches that feel hot to the touch with sharply defined borders are typical. Other types of skin cellulitis may have less sharply defined borders; red streaks, radiating from the patch, indicate the involvement of lymph vessels. Tissues of the floor of the mouth, the neck, the orbital socket, the pelvis and uterus are common targets for infection. Cellulitis of any form is potentially very dangerous. Treatment usually involves antibiotics and sulfonamides.

Numerous studies have demonstrated the effectiveness of centella triterpenes in the treatment of cellulitis.[29-32] For example, in one study, 48 of 65 patients, who had undergone other therapies without success, responded favorably (with complete healing) to the oral administration of centella during a 55 day test period. The investigators concluded that the product would also be useful in the treatment of many other ill-defined syndromes, such as those experienced by regular oral contraceptive users and other conditions that involve swelling in the lower limbs due to venous or lymphatic insufficiency.[29]

Perhaps the most extensive study to date examined the effects of centella on 477 patients, most of whom had already tried other products without success. Eighty per cent of these patients were healed with the centella extract.[32]

Venous Insufficiency /Phlebitis

Centella triterpenes have been examined for their effect on venous insufficiency, or the decrease in blood flow through the veins, a condition underlying several common ailments. The results have been uniformly positive, in the sense that significant improvement is observed in most cases. A wide range of individual manifestations of symptoms can be exhibited by people suffering from chronic venous insufficiency.

Using phlebitis as a model of venous insufficiency, investigators have attempted to pinpoint the action of centella more exactly in the hope of not only learning more about centella, but of discovering more about the body's healing processes themselves. For example, in one study centella was compared to two commonly used therapeutic agents considered to possess first, the ability to protect capillary stability and second, a capacity for stimulating capillary dynamic activity without inducing active expansion and contraction of the veins. Since centella triterpenes act at the level of connective tissue, the scientists were hoping to elucidate the role of connective tissue in microscopic circulatory dynamics. Patients suffering from phlebitis (the inflammation of the veins), due to prolonged confinement to bed, were used as subjects. Such confinement produces complicated changes in the relationship of veins to bones and joints that are thought to produce the inflammation. The centella extract produced the best results on all parameters, leading the authors to conclude not only that centella triterpenes were ideally suited for the treatment of manifestations of venous insufficiency that arise due to prolonged confinement, but to propose the revolutionary hypothesis that metabolic and biochemical factors contribute as much or more to the correction of confinement problems than do tensional and postural factors.[14]

Ranging in severity from mild to serious, phlebitis, is a common condition, especially in the veins of the lower limbs. If the inflammation occurs in a deep vein, the condition may have serious consequences. Phlebitis occurs most frequently where there is poor circulation due to some other condition, such as blood disorders, obesity, other infections, or prolonged confinement without exercise or frequent changes of position. It also occurs in about 1% of women after childbirth.

Because of its selective effects on connective tissue, centella has been highly successful in studies on its action relative to phlebitis and other examples of venous insufficiency. In one study, 72 per cent of 125 patients suffering from varices, phlebitis, capillary fragility and paraphlebitis, were successfully treated.[33] The success rate of other studies has ranged from 70 to 90 per cent.[34-39] In addition to the symptoms cited above, the following conditions have responded well to centella treatment: heaviness of the legs, tingling, and nocturnal cramps.[34]

The most recent studies have focused on the use of centella to treat persons with long standing or chronic venous insufficiency. In one study, an extract of centella, in tablet form, was administered to 26 female patients over a period of 30 days. Several indices were used to evaluate effectiveness: postural edema, alterations in observable health of skin, induced pain, nocturnal cramps, numbness and sensation of weight. The treatment induced a statistically significant remission of all symptoms, except the numbness and appearance of the skin.[35] In another study, tablets were given to 40 men and women with chronic venous insufficiency, for a period of 30 days. Centella was effective in ameliorating the symptoms of swelling or edema of the lower limbs, dilation of the blood vessels, health of skin, and ulcerative conditions.[36]

Conclusion

Taking all the research together, the most general conclusion we can make is that centella, mainly because of the presence of medically important triterpenes, has a clear and consistent healing effect on most, if not all, solid tissues of the body, including the skin, connective tissues, lymph tissues, blood vessels and mucous membranes. This product has found its most successful applications in the treatment of conditions involving, or based on, venous insufficiency, tissue inflammation and infection, and post surgical healing. It stimulates and accelerates the normal cellular repair processes, rather than instituting some artificial process.

Specific conditions that have been successfully treated with centella include skin sores, bed sores and ulcers, surgical incisions and tears, cellulitis, phlebitis, chronic venous insufficiency, varices, disorders of fat metabolism, leg cramps and edema.

Therapeutic Action.

Skin injuries

The clinical research has clearly specified some of the more important applications for centella triterpenes: open skin sores, wounds, tears, cuts and ulcers. Applied topically or taken internally, a centella extract should produce rapid and efficient healing of all variations in such conditions. It accomplishes these ends by directly stimulating the metabolic processes involved in the production of new skin tissue. It doesn't work by artificially stimulating cell division and proliferation, but by making sick cells well (through the production of proteins, lipids, etc.), so that they can respond to normal reproductive forces, etc.. This property is not restricted to structural cells, but applies with equal or greater force to connective tissues.

Confinement

A particularly important application of centella is in the treatment of problems commonly experienced by persons confined to bed, either in the hospital or at home; for bed sores or phlebitis, centella is the perfect solution. Though not always effective, it works in the vast majority of cases, and many doctors consider it the first line of defense. The mechanisms underlying the healing of bed sores are discussed above; for phlebitis, below.

Venous insufficiency

Poor circulation, because of inactivity or disease, may lead to additional problems. Centella nurtures the veins in several ways: by strengthening and repairing the connective and supporting tissues; by decreasing capillary fragility; by nutritively supporting the cells of the vein. Part of this process is rather indirect; it involves the nourishment of efferent (motor) neurons, whose task it is to stimulate growth and metabolism in peripheral organs and tissues.

The most significant manifestation of venous insufficiency is phlebitis or inflammation of the veins, particularly in the legs. A sometimes difficult condition to treat, phlebitis yields extremely well to centella treatment. Until the advent of centella, normal treatment rarely involved medication; it consisted mainly of arduous mechanical tasks, like excercise or, for bed-ridden patients, frequent repositioning. Daily administration of centella has dramatically reduced the need for mechancial stimulation, and improved the outlook for total recovery.

Cellulitis and other skin infections

Though not usually recognized as such, cellulitis occurs frequently in people. Many of the more severe infectious inflammations of the tissues just under the surface of the skin are of this type. Erysepilas is a common manifestation. Such inflammations often involve underlying nerves, and can lead to sclerosis. Blood poisoning is another common complication.

It is of major signifcance, therefore, that centella triterpenes have been found to be extremely effective in halting the course of cellulitic infections and in accelerating their healing. It follows that other, less severe, forms of skin infections are likely to yield to treatment with centella.

Other Applications

In addition to the above well-documented uses, we should not lose track of other less well-researched effects: nerve tonic and sedative; learning and memory stimulant; nourishing tonic, and so forth. We hope that these properties will eventually be investigated and verified.

Route of Administration.

In most of the early studies, centella asciaticosides and triterpenes were administered parenterally, that is either via injection in the muscle or directly into the infected skin area, or into a vein. Topical routes have also been used, as in the application of some kind of special impregnated gauze, bandage or ointment. The oral route was seldom used at first, but has increased in use during the last several years. The results of all methods of administration appear to be comparable. Which route one chooses is therefore usually more a matter of convenience than of efficacy.

Taken orally, tablet or capsule forms are both effective.

Dosage.

A good centella product should contain 25 mg of triterpenes to conform to the standards established in research trials. Two to four tablets or capsules per day is normally sufficient. As mentioned at the beginning of this chapter, I prefer, and highly recommend to others, that centella extract in a base of whole centella be used instead of a purified centella extract by itself.

Toxicity.

Centella asiacticosides and other triterpenes appear to be completely nontoxic. Both the whole plant and its active constituents are generally regarded as safe in countries throughout the world.

References.

1. Lythgoe, B., & Tripett, S. "Derivtives of *centella asiatica* used against leprosy," Centlloside. Nature, **163**, 259-260, 1949. and Boiteau, P., Buzas, A., Lederer, E., & Polonsky, J. "Derivatives of *centella asiatica* used against leprosy. Chemical constitution of asiaticoside." Nature, **163**, 258, 1949.
2. Heyne, K. De Nuttige Planten van Indonesie, 3rd Ed. Part I., pp. 1-1450; Part II., pp. 1451-1660; pp. I-CCXLCI. Wageningen, 1950.
3. Lepine, J. "De l'hydrocotlyle asiatica Linne," Journal Pharm. Chim., III, **28**, 47-59.
4. Boiteau, P., Buzas, A., Lederer, E. & Polonsky, J. "Sur la constitution chimique de l'asiaticoside, 'heteroside' naturel contre la lepre. Bull. Soc. Chim. Biol., **31**, 46-51, 1949.
5. Boiteau, P. & Saracino, R. "Premier essais au sujet de l'action de l'asiaticoside sur les lupus erythemateux et sur certains lesions produites par les bacilles de Hansen et Koch," Medecin Francais, **8**, 251, 1948.
6. Boiteau, P. &Ratsimamanga, A.R., "L'asiaticoside extrait de 'centella asiatica' et ses emplois therapeutiques dans la cicatrisation des plaies experimentales et rebelles (lepre, tuberculose et lupus)," Therapie, **11**, 125, 1956.
7. Lawrence, et. al. 1967
8. May, 1968
9. Del Vecchio, A., Senni, I., Cossu, G., & Molinaro, M. "Effetti della centella asiatica sull'attivita biosintetica di fibroblasti in coltura." Farmaco, Ed. Prague, **39**, 355, 1984.
10. Tincani and Troldi, 1962
11. Viala, A., Cano, J.P., Durand, A. Paulin, R., Roux, F., Placidi, M., Pinhas, Hl., Lefournier, C. "Etude chez l'animal du passage transcutane des principes actif de l'extrait titre de centella asiatica L. marques au tritium apres application sous forme de 'tulle gras' et 'd'onguent'." Therapie, **32**, 573, 1977.
12. Chasseaud, L.F., Fry, B.J., Hawkins, D.R., Lewis, J.D., Sword, I.P., & Taylor Hathway, D.E. "The metabolism of asiatic acid, madecassic acid and asiaticoside in the rat." Arzneimittel Forschung, **21**, 1379, 1971.
13. Hachen, A., & Bourgoin, J.Y. "Etude anatomo-clinique des effets de l'extrait titre de centella asiatica dans la lipodystrophie localisee." Med. Prat. #738-Suppl., 7, 1979.
14. Allegra, C. "Studio capillaroscopico comparativo tra alcuni bioflavonoidi e frazione totale triterpenica di centella asiatica nell'insufficienza venosa." Clin Ter., **110**, 555, 1984.
15. Boely, C, & Ratsimamanga, A.R. "Traitment des ulceres de jambe par l'extrait de 'centella madagascariensis'." Presse Med., **66**, 1933, 1958.
16. Farris, G. "L'azione terapeutica dell'asiaticoside in campo dermatologico." Minerva Med., **51**, 2244, 1960.
17. Fincato, M. "Sul trattamento di lesioni cutanee con estratto di 'centella asiatica'." Minerva Med., **15**, 1235, 1960.
18. Ugo, A. "L'asiaticoside in alcune affezioni della cute." Boll. Soc. Med. Chir., Varese., **15**, 145, 1960.
18a. Borsalino, G. "L'asiaticoside nella terapia di lesioni ulcerative traumatiche e varicose degli arti." Romagna Med., **14**, 335, 1962.
19. Maleville, J. "Etude clinique d'un nouveau tulle gras." Gaz. Med. It., **86**, 593, 1979.
20. Apperti, M., Senneca, H., Sito, G., Grasso, C., & Izzo, A., "Sperimentazione dell'estratto

di centella asiatica nelle ulcere trofiche e nei procesi riparativi tissutalli." Quad. Chir. Prat., 3, 115, 1982.

21. Remotti, G. & Colombo, P.A. "L'asiaticoside nella terapia delle lesioni cervicali di natura non neoplastica." Riv. Ost. Ginec. Prat., 44, 572, 1962.

22. Baudon-Glanddier, Brivady. "Lesion perineales et asiaticoside." Gaz. Med. France, 70, 2463, 1963.

23. Torre, Ph., Dannadieu, J.M., & Braditch, J.L. "Activite cicatrisante de l'asiaticoside dans les plaier obstetricales du perinee." Clinique, 58 (681), 203, 1963.

24. Chisale, E., Serra, G.E. & Rapallo, G.B., "L'azione terapeutica dell'asiaticoside su ectopie colposcopicamente diagnosticate." Min., Ginec., 13, 799, 1961.

25. Heller, L. "Madecassol en gynecologie." Gaz. Med. France, 32, 6626, 1968.

26. Castellani, L., Gillet, J.Y., Lavernhe, G., & Dellenbach, P. "Asiaticoside et cicatrisation del episiotomies." Bull. Ped. Soc. Gynec. Obstet. Franc., 18, 184, 1966.

27. Pignataro, O., & Teatini, G.P. "Ricera clinica sull'azione cicatrizzante del madecassol nei confronti della mucosa orofaringea." Minera Med., 56, 2683, 1965.

28. Colonna d'Istria, J., & Savy, P. "Recherche sur l'action cicatrisante du madecassol en chirurgie cervicale et laryngee, apres radiations." J.F.O.R.L., 19, 507, 1970.

29. Dalloz-Bourguignon, A. "Etude de l'action de l'extrait titre de centella asiatica (a propos de 65 observations rercuillies en clientele privee)." Gaz. Med. France, 82, 4579, 1975.

30. Bargheon, J. "Cellulite et centella asiatica." Vie Med., 57, 597, 1976.

31. Bailly, P.J. "Une nouvelle therapeutique de la cellulite par l'extrait de centella asiatica." Med Prat., (629), 37, 1976.

32. Cezes, A. & Combalie, J.C. "477 cas de cellulite traites par madecassol." J. Med Esthetique, 3, (12), 31, 1976.

33. Frileux, C., & Cope, R. "Etude d'une nouvelle medication du tissue conjonctif veineux: l'extrait titre de centella asiatica." Gaz Med France, 78, 5052, 1971.

34. Boely, C. "Indications therapeutiques de l'extrait titre de centella asiatica en phlebologie.' Gaz. Med. France, 82, 741, 1975.

35. Pastore, A., & Zorzoli, C., "Terapia medica della I.V.C.: la centella asiatica (sperimentazione in doppio cieco vs/placebo." Clin. Europ., 20, 910, 1981.

36. Mazzola, M., & Gini, M.M. "La centella asiatica nella terapia della insufficienza venos cronica. Ricerca clinica controllata a cecita doppia vs placebo." Clin. Europ., 21, 160, 1982.

37. Cappelli, R. "Studio farmacologico clinico sull'effetto dell'estratto titolato di centella asiatica nell'insufficienza venosa cronica degli arti inferori." Giorn. It. Angiol., 3, 44, 1983.

38. Mariani, G. & Patuzzo, E. "Il trattamento dell'insufficienza venosa con estratto di centella asiatica." Clin. Europ., 22, 154, 1983.

39. Allegra, C. "Studio capillaroscopico comparativo tra alcuni bioflavonoidi e frazione totale treterpenica di centella asiatica nell'insufficienza venosa.

40.

41. Mowrey, D.B., "Capsicum, Ginseng and Gotu Kola in combination," The Herbalist, Premier Issue, 22-28, 1975.

42. Ramaswamy, A.S., Periyasamy, S.M. & Basu, N. Journal of Research in Indian Medicine, 4, 160-175, 1970.

Echinacea
(echinacea angustifolia, echinacea purpurea)

For The Immune System

Guaranteed Potency Constituents.

Echinacosides in *purpurea* (*angustifolia* is standarized against a "fingerprint" of purported active constituents). The last 30 years' research has identified the echinacoside glycosides as comprising the primary antibiotics in *echinacea purpurea.* But it would be a big mistake at this point in time to use a pure echinacoside extract. There are many other biologically active substances in echinacea, and there is evidence that they work synergistically. The polysaccharides, for example, possess the best immune stimulating properties and are also antiviral. Other constituents have been shown to possess good anti-tumor, bacteriostatic, and anesthetic activity. Currently, only the echinacosides can be standardized and guaranteed at a certain level. However, the general feeling is that, if the echinacosides are present, then so are the polysaccharides and other constituents. The best approach, for the present, is to standardize the level of echinacosides in *purpurea*, so as to guarantee a product with a reliable degree of activity, but to leave these in a base of whole herb extract. This is particularly important in a market flooded with echinacea products of questionable worth. As for *angustifolia*, standardization according to the presence and concentration of any single constituent has not yet been achieved. The "fingerprint" method produces a product of excellent quality. Mixtures of *purpurea* and *angustifolia* are also possible.

We hope that in the future, other constituents in echinacea will be standardized and guaranteed. Until that becomes possible, an echinacoside-Guaranteed Potency echinacea has the best chance of having adequate levels of all active constituents.

History.

Since echinacea grew abundantly throughout North American prairies, plains, and open woodlands, it would have been hard for the Amerindians to have overlooked this valuable plant. And they didn't.

In fact, ethnobotanical research has revealed literally scores of ways echinacea was used by the tribes of the plains and woods.

It is quite natural that the great interest in echinacea demonstrated in Amerindian and early colonial folklore would arouse the curiosity of physicians. European physicians had already made considerable progress in applying echinacea in the treatment of fevers and infections, but it would be decades before their science would begin a systematic investigation of the plant.

Meanwhile, American eclectic physicians utilizing whatever poor instrumentation they had, enthusiastically pursued research studies on echinacea. And in many ways, American research conducted during this period was far superior to that of the Europeans. Both orthodox physicians and scientists (e.g. Lloyd and King), as well as the most authoritative eclectics (Felter and Ellingwood), agreed that echinacea had true medicinal potential, especially against infections, snake bites and cancer. But, they weren't entirely of one mind regarding how the herb worked. Their explanations ran the gamut, from blood purifier to, "the revitalization of tissue," to "a corrector of the depravation of the body's fluids," to "organizer of the defensive powers of the system."

Perhaps the best work was done by Victor von Unruh in 1915–1916, who actually looked at the effects of the plant on blood cultures and made hundreds of careful blood counts. He wrote that

> "Echinacea increases the phagocytic power of the leukocytes; it normalizes the percentage count of neutrophiles. . . . Hyper-leukocytosis and leukopenia are directly improved by echinacea; the proportion of white to red blood cells is rendered normal; and the elimination of waste products is stimulated to a degree that puts this drug in first rank among all alteratives. . . . The leukocytes are directly stimulated by Echinacea, their activity is increased, the percentage among the different classes of neutrophiles is rendered normal, and phagocytosis is thus raised to its best functioning capacity."

All of which means that echinacea normalizes the white blood cell count and stimulates intracellular processes that destroy pathogens such as viruses and bacteria.[1] Von Uhruh was talking about the immune system long before orthodox medicine had recognized the importance of it.

Eclectic physicians, during this time, used echinacea in the treatment of typhoid, meningitis, malaria, diphtheria, boils, carbuncles, abscesses, snake, animal and insect bites, uremic poisoning, canker sores, appendicitis, cholera, erysipelas, cancer, bed sores, syphilis, tetanus, impetigo, and even rabies. It was used to counteract fever (lower the temperature), ward off infection, stimulate sweating, the flow of saliva and the appetite, stimulate blood flow, increase kidney and liver action, stimulate digestion and assimilation, improve nutrition, stimulate the lymphatic system, prevent auto-intoxication, restore the balance in bodily fluids, subdue delirium, and reduce the pulse.

Reports from that era resound with enthusiasm and excitement. Eclectic physicians sustained intense interest, both therapeutic and scientific, in echinacea for as long as they could, hoping that the medical revolution, then in its infancy, would incorporate echinacea into its bag of remedies. But, in spite of those hopes and efforts, a couple of early governmental screening tests, which failed to substantiate the claims being made for echinacea, was all it took to irreversibly diminish the interest of the orthodox medical and scientific communities.[2]

Later, in Germany, in keeping with that country's commitment to the systematic and thorough investigation of folklore medicine, great strides in research began in 1950 and have continued into the present era. The bulk of the studies reviewed below can be credited to German interest in echinacea.

Method of Action.

Most of what is scientifically known about echinacea has been learned in basic laboratory research. Good clinical studies are few and far between. The primary emphasis of this chapter will, therefore, be on mechanisms of action. The Therapeutic Research section will contain what little clinical work is available. And in the Therapeutic Action section we will attempt to extrapolate from data in this section to show how echinacea should be used in daily life.

It should be remembered that most, maybe all, of the properties of echinacea discussed in this section, in one way or another, contribute to improved immune system functioning.

Antibiotic action

Glycosides, isolated from the roots of echinacea, have been shown to have mild antibiotic activity against streptococci and staphylococcus aureus; the main active glycoside was identified as echinacoside.[3-4] About 6 mg of echinacoside was equivalent to one unit of penicillin.

It has been found that another constituent of echinacea, echinacin, may be a more effective antibiotic than cortisone. For example, streptococcal infection spreads rapidly in guinea pigs pretreated with cortisone, but is contained by echinacin. It has also been found that 0.04 ml of fresh plant extract possesses a hyaluronidase inhibitory action (see below) equal to 1 mg of cortisone.[5-7]

A Polish study found that a simple echinacea tincture was able to reduce both the rate of growth and the rate of reproduction in the common vaginal infectious protozoon, *Trichomonas vaginalis*.[8]

Another common vaginal infection is caused recurrently by the yeast *candida albicans*. In one of the few clinical studies done to date, echinacea was found to be effective in halting the recurrence of this infection.[9]

Connective tissue stabilization

In recent years, research has discovered one of the mechanisms by which echinacea prevents infection and repairs tissue damaged by infection, particularly of a viral nature. One of the main actions of echinacea is to inhibit the activity of the enzyme *hyaluronidase*. One of the primary defense mechanisms of the body is known as the *hyaluronidase system* (H-system). It involves the ability of connective "ground" substance, or hyaluronic acid (HA) to act as a barrier against the intrusion of pathogenic organisms into the tissues of the body). Picture HA as a bowl of jello in which cells are suspended, like little white marshmallows. Picture germs bouncing off the surface of the jello, like kids on a trampoline. As long as the jello is firm, nothing can get at the marshmallows. But picture germs with teeth somehow grabbing hold of the jello surface, somehow activating an enzyme in the HA— hyaluronidase — which otherwise, just seems to float around in the HA with nothing to do. Germ-activated, hyaluronidase goes quickly to work, as if making up for lost time, punching holes in the HA. Picture the bowl of jello slowly turning to water as the system becomes leaky. Finally, picture the invading pathogens, attaching themselves to exposed cell surfaces, penetrating and killing the cell. This microscopic process is observable to the naked eye as inflammation.

As mentioned, echinacea inhibits hyaluronidase; it does so by combing with the enzyme, thereby inactivating it. The result is a temporary increase in the integrity of the HA barrier. Fewer pathogens are able to stimulate the destruction of the ground substance. The health of the body is maintained, even when exposed to the germ-ridden environmental conditions present during cold and flu season. The ability of echinacea, and other plants, to inhibit the inflammatory response may well rest on this anti-hyaluronidase action. The constituent in echinacea, responsible for inhibiting hyaluronidase, has been identified as a very complex polysaccharide called echinacin B.[10-12] However, there are indications that non-polysaccharide substances (isobutylamides and polyines) may also be involved in the mechanism just described.

Interestingly, a mechanism very similar to the H-system has been proposed as a possible substrate for the generation of rheumatism and tumor formation and the beginnings of cancer.[13]

Connective tissue repair

The anti-hyaluronidase activity of echinacea has also been shown to be involved in the regeneration of cellular connective (granulomatous) tissue destroyed during infection and in the elimination of pathogenic organisms creating the infection. In one study, heterogeneous and homogeneous fibrin grafts (under the influence of leucocytic enzymes) were transformed, via amino acids, into components of the connective tissue substance. In other words, the stuff (fibrin) that the body uses to form blood clots was grafted into wounds, so it would take root and accelerate the production of new skin tissue in the area of the wound. Compared to pure fibrin grafts, echinacea-treated fibrin grafts exhibited increased healing tendency of the wound areas and less marked leukocytic infiltration. New fibrocytes appeared more rapidly and on a larger scale, and the extract appeared to possess significant protective action towards the new tissue (mucopolysaccharides) being produced by the fibrocytes in the mesoderm layer of the skin. The mesoderm (the layer between the ectoderm and the entoderm) is responsible for the production of all types of connective tissue, as well as bone marrow, blood, and lymph. Enhanced protection of this layer, therefore, helps to ensure rapid and effective healing. To summarize, echinacea stimulates the breakdown of fibrin into mucopolysaccharides, which are transformed into new connective tissue by the young fibroblasts, the formation of which is also stimulated by echinacea.[14-16]

At this point the reader may wish to review the manner in which centella stimulates the repair of connective tissues (see pages 34-35). It will be seen that the actions of echinacea and centella complement one another very nicely. But whereas centella is concerned with overall strength and integrity of the connective tissues, echinacea's role appears to be more concerned with cellular systems involved in the natural defense of the body to infectious organisms.

Macrophage and T-cell activity

The immune system, as far as we understand it, appears to be composed of several armies of highly organized chemicals, all acting together in extremely intricate ways in order to intercept and defeat a rag tag group of invading substances, including toxins, bacteria, viruses, dying tissue, allergens, antigens, clotting blood and a motley crew of waste materials.

I. *White Blood Cells*. aka *leukocytes*. Cells that circulate in the blood stream in search of invaders to have for lunch; they squeeze out into the interstitial fluid (stuff between cells) when summoned to a site of invasion.

   A. *Phagocytes*. aka *granulocytes*. White blood cells whose primary job it is to engulf the invaders. The phagocytes respond to invasion in a non-specific manner, simply attacking everything of a foreign nature that is in sight. They respond to the summons of chemical messengers produced when invaders breach the body's defenses, exploding mast cells and releasing histamine and other messengers into the blood (inflammatory response).

   1. *neutrophils*. Tiny, short-lived cells, stored in the bone marrow by the billions, released in response to infection; these are the foot--soldiers, or 'grunts' of the immunological army. Throwing themselves into the foray, they die by the billions. They contain enzyme-filled granules in their cytoplasm. After engulfing an invader the granules empty their powerful enzymes, which kill the invader; after destroying a few invaders, the neutrophil succumbs to its own enzymes. Neutrophils are incapable of reproduction. The targets of the neutrophils are primarily micro-organisms.

   2. *eosinophils*. These specialized cells devote their existence to the devouring of IgE-antibody-allergen complexes. Eosinophils are an intrinsic part of the allergic reaction.

   3. *monocytes*. Circulating in the blood, these small cells are relatively powerless recruits, but once summoned to the site of battle they quickly transform into huge, powerful marines capable of enormous destructive power; in this form they are known as macrophages. As such, their appetite is unsatiable. These may live for years, and are capable of fusing together in order to defeat a particularly large foe. The macrophage counterpart to the granule is the lysosome, also containing potent enzymes. Capable of reproduction, the number of circulating macrophages can become very large during the heat of the battle. Macrophages destroy micro-organisms; likewise, they engulf ineffective red blood cells, dead and dying tissue, exhausted neutrophils, and other debris — even indigestible material.

   B. *Basophils*. White blood cells that do not devour other materials, but play an important role in inflammation and the allergic response. IgE-basophil-antigen interactions lead to the acceleration of the body's defense system.

   C. *Lymphocytes*. White blood cells involved in the body's specific immune system. The guided missiles. Lymphocytes seem to congregate in the lymph system, especially the lymph nodes. The lymph system is a kind of secondary circulatory system with channels that flow throughout the body. Large lymphatic ducts empty into the blood stream near the heart. Substances such as oxygen, food, fluids, white blood cells and so forth leave the blood stream and make their way to individual tissue, organ and muscle cells via the lymphatic tissue and finally enter the blood stream for further processing by the liver, kidneys, and other organs. The lymphatic system collects bacteria and other invaders and carries them to special lymphatic tissues such as the spleen, tonsils, lymph nodes, adenoids and bone marrow. Individual lymphocytes are genetically programmed to attack very specific targets. Young lymphocytes are undifferentiated, but eventually develop into two major classes. Any substance that elicits activity from lymphocytes is called an antigen.

　　　　1. *B lymphocytes*. (B-cells) These produce proteins called antibodies (gamma globulins or immunoglobulins) which have very specific targets. When some B-cells and antigens meet, the B-cell transforms itself into a plasma cell which goes into mass production of antibodies (2,000/second!). Other B-cells transform into rapidly multiplying memory cells which circulate throughout the body preparing it for the next encounter with the antigen. Long-lived. Antibodies are short-lived.

　　　　a. *IgA*. Found mainly in mucous membranes. Intercepts antigens in nose and throat.

　　　　b. *IgD*. Not much known about the role of this antibody.

　　　　c. *IgE*. Binds to certain antigens to cause allergic reactions. Attaches to basophils and similar cells called mast cells. When they encounter an antigen, configuration changes cause the mast cell to explode, dumping histamine, enzymes, etc. into the blood which, in turn, attract distant immune system troops to the site of battle.

　　　　d. *IgG*. Most common antibody. Extremely important for proper immune system functioning.

　　　　e. *IgM*. Largest antibody. Also very important in immune system functioning.

　　　　2. *T lymphocytes*. (T-cells) These long-lived cells also transform into active and memory cells when they encounter an antigen. T- cells are actually the body's main defense against acute bacterial infection; they also destroy fungi, cancerous cells, transplanted tissue, wounded cells harboring viruses and bacteria, etc. T-cells are also important in stimulating the production of B-cells. T-cells produce substances called lymphokienes that draw macrophages, neutrophils and eosinophils toward sensitized T-cells, signal them to remain at the site

of the battle, activate the macrophages to incredible activity, inhibit the reproducibility of viruses, affect the clotting of blood and so forth.

    a. *Killer T-cells*. These attack target antigens directly, killing one and moving on to the next.

    b. *Helper T-cells*. These activate B-cells, causing the appropriate ones to transform into plasma cells and flood the blood stream with antibodies.

    c. *Suppressor T-cells*. These are responsible for keeping the whole system from running amok. They monitor and adjust the level of antibodies and counteract the action of Helper T-cells.

II. *The Complement System*. When an antibody binds to an antigen another secondary, or complementary set of chemical reactions is initiated. The binding activates the complement proteins in the blood stream. This set of nine proteins (C1 - C9) are transformed into active enzymes which attach to the surface of the invader and essentially burn a hole through the cell membrane causing the cell to explode. The C1 protein is actually a group of related proteins often called the *properdin* proteins. Other complement proteins directly attack viruses; others attach to antigens and make them a more susceptible target for phagocytes; some complement proteins may act as phagocytes themselves. The complement system thus plays an important role in the immune reaction.

    Summary. What happens, then, in a typical invasion is something like the following. Invading micro-organisms first encounter whatever quantity of macrophages, neutrophils, B and T cells might be present in the immediate vicinity. The battle is enjoined, but the defense is not sufficient to win. The activation of basophils releases histamine; destruction of phagocytes produces other chemical messengers — inflammation is initiated and a flood of chemical signals are sent to bone marrow where the production of phagocytes is increased. More macrophages, neutrophils and lymphocytes are drawn to the site of invasion. Meanwhile, any antibodies at the battle lock onto predestined foes, and the complement system is brought into action. The complement system directly kills some invaders, makes others more susceptible to attack from phagocytes, and holds the ground until the reserves arrive. Debris from the complement system battle also produces strong attracting signals for phagocytes and lymphocytes. With the arrival of T-cells the skirmishes elevate into wholesale war. The killer T-cells attack antigens directly, and T-cells begin to produce the lymphokienes which serve to intensify the battle. The war thus begins (excuse this extended metaphor) as a clash between the body's sentinels and the environment's guerilla forces at limited sites of invasion, and escalates to full-scale battle raging on fronts throughout the body. Medics, scouts, messengers, command posts, officers, non-coms, grunts, reserves, even chaplins — they're all there. Eventually, usually, the good guys win, but not without tremendous cost. How well you or I or any other person does depends upon hundreds of intricate, lablile, mutually dependent, biochemical, genetic and physiological factors. The whole system is only as strong as its weakest link.

Using the above abbreviated account of the immune system for reference, the actions of echinacea may now be explored more intelligibly

Purified polysaccharides prepared from echinacea possess a strong activating force on the body's macrophage-mediated defense system. The large macrophages initiate the destruction of harmful micro-organisms and pathogens that cause bacterial and viral infections and cancer. The process is called phagocytosis and depends not only on the cytotoxic activity of macrophages but on other cells such as the T-cell lymphocytes, which produce molecules that activate macrophages. Echinacea has been found capable of activating the macrophages by itself; this action appears to be independent of any cooperative effect with T-lymphocytes. (In fact, in several related tests, echinacea was unable to stimulate T-lymphocytes at all.) Once activated, macrophages respond in the normal manner by developing high lethality toward cancerous target cells The macrophages, activated by echinacea, are also instrumental in the production and secretion of interleukin 1 and B lymphocytes.[17-18] Researchers point out that one of the advantages of using echinacea to stimulate macrophage activity is that, unlike most drugs used for this purpose, echinacea is completely non-toxic.

In other studies, polysaccharides were discovered that did stimulate T-cell activity — in fact T-cell activity increased twenty to thirty percent more than when another very strong T-cell stimulator was used.[19-20] Since differing preparations of echinacea were used in these studies, the contradictions in results regarding T-lymphocyte stimulation are not unreasonable. However, at this time the problem has not been resolved.

Cancer

The same purified extract, referred to above, produces a pronounced extracellular cytotoxic activity against tumor target cells. USDA researchers have also discovered a tumor-inhibiting principle in echinacea, this one being an oncolytic lipid-soluble hydrocarbon from the essential oil. Tumors inhibited were Walker's carcinosarcoma and lymphocytic leukemia.[21]

Based on everything else we know about its action, we can suppose that echinacea fights cancerous growth by stimulating the production of key lymphocytes which in turn trigger the activation of cells, such as the natural killer cells, that destroy the cancer cells.

Direct anti-inflammatory activity

A German patent revealed the presence of two factors, A & B in echinacea. Factor A caused stress and fever, while factor B had an anti--hyaluronidase effect. The two factors appeared to be somewhat offsetting and this study served to underscore the complexities involved in plant chemistry, especially when introduced to living organisms. Interestingly, the author's main intent, apparently successful, was to produce a substance that could be recommended for the detoxification of medicines and other remedies and would be appropriate for use in prolonging the amount of time medicines actively circulate in the blood, by delaying their resorption.[22]

Fraction B was fundamentally effective in the wound healing process, as evidenced by the production of fibrous scar tissue in the wound. Other researchers have reasoned that the active principles in the echinacea extract actually combined, somehow, with hyaluronic acid to produce a complex that was resistant to attack by hyaluronidase and that not only restricted the diffusion of viruses in the wound, but facilitated the regeneration of fibrous connective tissues.[23-24]

Other researchers investigated the anti-inflammatory properties of echinacea, using the standard carrageenan and croton oil tests. In the first test inflammation is caused by injecting carrageenan under the skin of the hind paw of rats. This quickly induces edema. Echinacina B significantly prevented the inflammation and swelling from occurring. In the second test inflammation is caused by rubbing croton oil on the ears of mice. This creates a measurable and reliable inflammatory response that was significantly inhibited by echinacina B. Though the echinacea extract was effective in all stages of the carrageenan-induced inflammatory response, which is mediated by histamine, 5–HT, kinins and the metabolites of arachidonic acid, it appeared to be most potent in the later phases; the later stages are reportedly characterized by the release of prostaglandins from medium-sized phagocytic neutrophils, after their interaction with carrageenan. The dermatitis induced by irritant croton oil is reportedly mediated also by arachidonic acid metabolites, released during the later stages of the phlogistic process.[25]

Properdin

With the discovery of a substance called properdin, the whole question of natural resistance to disease entered a new arena. The idea of the complement system, whose role was to activate mechanisms that would destroy bacteria and viruses, had been talked about for many years, but there was not much evidence to support the concept. Attempts to attribute the natural resistance of the body to one or another factor in the blood or some organ led ultimately to confusing contradictions. It looked for awhile like a thorough, experimentally-based analysis of the complement was impossible.

Then properdin was discovered. It provided the necessary link and opened the door to decades of fruitful research. Through the observation of this chemical's rise and fall, production and destruction, activity and inactivity, much has been learned, and much more has been discovered. We still do not know all there is to know about properdin and the related complement proteins, but it is now certain these naturally occurring chemicals are intrinsically involved in the body's natural resistance to viral and bacterial infection, as discussed above.

Since echinacea had been shown to be involved in the hyaluronidase system, and since properdin and hyaluronic acid had been empirically connected, it was reasonable to study the relationship, if any, between echinacea and properdin. The results were startling; properdin levels, under the influence of echinacea (i.v. injections of 0.6 ml/kg in rabbits), sank a little at first, but then came back and zoomed to significantly greater levels than normal.[26-27]

Interferon induction

Interferon is another protein produced naturally within the body. While studies have shown that injections of interferon can have both good and bad effects on the body, most scientists agree that the stimulation of the body's interferon-producing systems may be responsible for increasing the body's natural defenses against infection and cancer.

One of the most intriguing studies on echinacea was done in Germany, in 1978. Researchers pretreated cells from human and mouse tissues with echinacin, and then infected them with influenza, herpes, and vesicular stomatitis (canker sore) viruses. This little petri dish study is a standard tool for determining the ability of substances to prevent infection and/or affect the course of infection. Comparative data from virtually hundreds of thousands of such studies is available; this greatly simplifies the task of categorizing agents according to their actions. In this case, however, the researchers were faced with the tedious and difficult task of differentiating between phagocytosis-induced and nonphagocytosis-induced healing processes. Greatly simplified, the results of the study were as follows: a 4–6 hour pre-treatment with echinacea increased the cells' resistance to subsequent infection by 50 to 80 percent, and maintained that resistance for the next 48 hours. These significant results align very nicely with those observed when interferon is used in the pretreatment phase.

Intrigued by these results, the researchers hypothesized that echinacea works in one way by stimulating T–cell lymphocytes, which, in turn, produce interferon, and in another way through cell surface chemistry, perhaps involving hyaluronidase.[28] This hypothesis has been disputed by other investigators, who maintain that the action of echinacea can be explained more simply as follows: the polysaccharides (and other chemicals) in echinacea actively compete with viruses for the receptor sites on cell membrane surfaces.[29] Whoever gets there first, wins. Such mechanisms usually operate in a kind of lock and key manner, but the exact mechanism in this case is still unknown. The idea that echinacea stimulates T–lymphocytes has been disputed empirically also (see discussion in the section on Macrophages and T–cells).

Summary/Immune system

Summarizing the properties of echinacea relative to the immune system, the following general statements pertain. On the most simple level, echinacea prevents and cures various kinds of bacterial and viral infections. One of its best known cellular actions is the inhibition of the enzyme hyaluronidase which, when activated, destroys the cementing, "ground," substance between cells, thereby allowing pathogens to infiltrate the body.

On a little more complex level, echinacea activates macrophages (and, perhaps, T–cells) that destroy cancerous cells and foreign intracellular invaders. It increases the level of phagocytosis in other ways, such as mediating the level of white blood cells such as the neutrophils, monocytes, eosinophils, and B lymphocytes. And, it has a profound effect on properdin levels, an indication that the complement system has been activated.

Perhaps the most complicated mechanisms under study are those involving the stimulation of interferon and/or interferon-like activity. Teasing these actions apart will be the work of decades.

There are still other ways by which echinacea may boost the body's immune system that are currently being investigated. For example, there are indications that the herb delays resorption of other drugs, thereby prolonging their action in the body. It could likewise prolong the effects of other herbs administered simultaneously.

Therapeutic Research.

As mentioned above, there has not been a lot of clinical data generated on echinacea during the era of modern medicine. The main reason for that has been the lack of a consensus relative to the total activity of the herb. As long as there remain mechanisms of action that cannot be completely ascertained in animal studies, pharmaceutical companies and university departments are reluctant to involve humans too much in research. In view of the remarkable properties of echinacea and its total lack of observed toxicity, the reluctance to proceed with clinical studies is, in this case, difficult to understand.

In one of the few attempts to quantify, or at least record, the action of echinacea on bacterial skin infections in humans, in recent times, German scientists reported that echinacea produced a rapid and complete restoration of skin tissue. The author attributed the effect to the acceleration of phagocytosis rate in the area of the infection.[30]

Another study purportedly found that echinacea stimulated the production of white blood cells in the bone marrow of patients undergoing radiology treatment.[31]

Recently, in a very good clinical study, 203 patients, who had been experiencing recurrent vaginal candida infections for several months, were treated with either an echinacea cream, or with a liquid extract plus the cream. The treatments were administered in a double--blind, cross-over manner. Every six months for two-three years, the patients were monitored to determine if there had been a recurrence of the infection. The results showed that the combination of treatments was by far the most effective in preventing recurrences. The application of just the cream was less than one-third as effective as the combined effects of cream plus extract.[32] More significantly, perhaps, than the results of this study, is the fact that the study was done at all. I predict that it signals the beginning of a new age in the study of echinacea, an age in which clinical research will proliferate.

It is impossible to discount the hundreds of case histories that have come to us, through the usually carefully controlled clinical research of the American eclectic physicians. The eclectics were very active from the late 1800's right up until the 1940's, after which not much was heard from them. During the height of eclectic activity, literally hundreds of cases were reported, in which echinacea was used to prevent and treat an incredible variety of infectious diseases: smallpox, typhoid, tetanus, diphtheria, syphilis, influenza, tuberculosis, yellow fever, malaria, polio, measles, rubella, whooping cough, mumps, cholera, the common cold, intestinal disease, etc. The herb was not always effective, and some eclectics were more successful than others in applying it. Some physicians were careful to do basic test-tube kinds of research. The resulting research reports, taken as a whole, overwhelmingly support the efficacy of echinacea over a wide range of conditions.[33-36] In fact, it is eclectic research that gave the impetus to modern European research interest in echinacea.

In a sense, the eclectics were way ahead of their time. Certainly, their understanding of the immune system anticipated modern conceptualizations, even though the body of knowledge they had to work with did not even closely approximate what we now know (but see below), and many of the terms have that quaint ring of folklore and ancient medicine (e.g., cholagogue, blood purifier, etc. — note, however the zeitgeist pop quaintness of some of our own expressions, e.g., adaptogen, immune-system stimulant, psycho-stimulant). Rather than invent new medicine, the eclectics were busy counting white blood cells; they understood, better than schools of orthodox medicine of the time, how to examine the relationships between white blood cell activity and therapeutic agents.

The eclectics ultimately lost the battle with orthodox medicine, not because their systems were any less sound than orthodoxy (in many ways they were vastly superior, less intrusive, gentler, and more effective), but because the latter was faster picking up the harsh but powerful drugs. Wedded to scientific achievement, modern medicine quickly adopted the one germ-one disease model and began to ignore wholistic concepts. Now that the one germ-one disease model has about played out, wholistic doctine and the vision of the eclectics are being rediscovered (and renamed, of course), especially with regard to the treatment of non-specific diseases, cancer, senility, Alzheimer's disease, AIDS, auto-immune disorders, and so forth.

Therapeutic Action.

Most of the actions of echinacea can all be related, in currently popular jargon, to proper immune system functioning. In times of stress, in harsh environments or seasons, whenever the body is in need of reinforcement, echinacea may supply the boost required to maintain the natural lines of resistance, to mend injured tissue, and to stimulate healthy body functioning.

Since the invention of the vaccination, we do not need echinacea to prevent or treat many of the world's most deadly infections. However, the common cold, yearly influenza outbreaks, childhood earaches, mild and moderate infections of all kinds are still the province of echinacea — anything, in fact that involves some kind of immune deficiency. We have found that echinacea beneficially affects many of the substrates of cellular immunity, and future research is bound to find more such mechanisms. Meanwhile, we will find that more conditions than cancer can be viewed in terms of the immune system, and we will learn even more about how to prevent breakdowns in this system. Echinacea, and other medicinal plants, are certain to play a central role in these developments.

As I study what is currently known about the immune system, I find more and more reason to want to put that phrase in quotes: "the immune-system," just as I currently insist on putting quotes around the term "adaptogen." Could these be simple catch-all phrases, labels that give an illusion of understanding to things little-comprehended? In studying echinacea, I find that its actions help put the immune system in perspective. Though much is known about the action of echinacea, there is still much that is not known about this plant. And it is precisely this unknown area that serves so nicely to put the whole adaptogen/immune stimulant/anti-everything dilemma in perspective. Will the adaptogenic double talk really turn out to be better understood as a function of proper immune system functioning? And what is "immune system functioning"? For that matter, what is the immune system itself? It is already an oversimplified, short-hand, phrase for a whole host of individual actions emanating from all of the body's functional systems. And what about all the little anti's? Antibiotic, anti-inflammatory, antirheumatic, antitoxin, anti-this, anti-that. Are not these also simply abbreviated terms for complicated processes that, when completely understood, won't be anti-anything?

The future?
Over 80 years ago, an eclectic physician wrote:

> "Nature has probably destined echinacea to be used for remedial purposes only, as a sustainer of vitality, an organizer of the defensive powers of the system, to such an extent as to be justly crowned the greatest immunizing agent in the entire vegetable kingdom, as far as is known to medical science."[37]

That is a bright vision, one we are seeing fulfilled.

Route of Administration.

There are several forms in which echinacea can be taken, including liquid extracts, syrups, ointments and tablets. The guaranteed potency echinacea is currently available only as a capsule. Taken orally, echinacea exhibits all of its reported beneficial properties. But ointments, used topically to treat candida infections, for example, may potentiate the action of the extract.

Dosage.

Guaranteed potency preparations of *echinacea purpurea* will contain 3.5% echinacosides. 125 mg capsules are standard. Daily intake should be restricted to what is deemed necessary. During cold and flu season, two to four capsules per day is sufficient. In the presence of acute infection, that dosage may be increased, without danger, to more than 8 capsules. In the presence of chronic infections, such as chronic hepatitis, echinacea may be used continuously for several months. However, for the maintenance of a healthy immune system, echinacea is most wisely used periodically — a few weeks on, and a few weeks off, throughout the year. Echinacea is not a tonic in all aspects; granted that it has been observed to stabilize the production of neutrophils, such tonic action has not been observed on other immune factors, such as properdin production. In the absence of conclusive experimental findings, it is both safe and wise to assume that the constant, unremitting use of echinacea could be stressful on certain aspects of the immune system. During breaks, the immune system will adapt and increase in natural strength.

The above recommendations accord with suggestions made by European manufacturers. As an immune system stimulant a daily quantity of 500 to 1000 mg (2-4 capsules) is recommended by most European manufacturers and physicians. Substantially more is recommended for the treatment of acute infections, inflammation and fever. Exceedingly large doses are said to contribute little, if any, positive activity beyond what can be achieved with moderate doses.

Toxicity.

Echinacea does not appear to be toxic even at very large doses.[38]

Incidentally, heavy use of echinacea may induce temporary infertility in the male. Hyaluronidase is one of three enzymes attached to the acrosomal membrane located on the head of the male spermatozoon. This enzyme attacks the intercellular matrix of the cumulus oophorus and clears a path to the zona pelucida, without which action the spermatozoon cannot bind to the zona and fertilization cannot take place. It would not be unreasonable to think, therefore, that men taking large amounts of echinacea would experience reduced fertility.[39]

References.

1. Felter, H.W. The Eclectic Materia Medica, Pharmacology and Therapeutics, Eclectic Medical Publications, Portland, Oregon, 1983 (first published in 1922).
2. Council on Pharmacy and Chemistry. 1090. "Echinacea considered valueless." Journal of the American Medical Association, 53(22), 1836.
3. Stoll, A., Renz, A. & Brack, A. "Antibacterial substances II. Isolation and constitution of echinacoside, a glycoside from the roots of echinacea augustifolia." Helvetic chimica acta, 33, 1877-1893, 1950.
4. Becker, V.H. "Against snakebites and influenza; use and components of echinacea angustifolia and e. purpurea." Deutsche Apotheker Zeitung, 122(45), 2020-2323, 1982.
5. Koch, E. & Uebel, H. "Experimental studies concerning the local action of echinacea purpurea on tissues." Arzneimittel-Forschung, 3, 16-19, 1953.
6. Koch, E. & Hasse, H. "A modification of the spreading test in animal assays." Arzneimittel-Forschung, 2, 454-467, 1952.
7. Koch, E. & Uebel, H. "Experimental studies on the local influence of cortisone and echinacin upon tissue resistance against streptococcus infection." Arzneimittel-Forschung, 4, 424-426, 1954.
8. Samochowiec, E., Urbanska, L, Manka, W. & Stolarska, E. "Ocen dzialania wyciagow calendula officinalis i echinacea angustifolia na trichomonas vaginalis in vitro." Wiadomosci Parzytologiczne, 25(1), 77-81, 1979.
9. Coeuginiet, E. "Recurrent candidiasis: adjuvant immunotherapy with different formulations of echinacin." Therapiewoche, 36(33), 33520-03358, 1986.
10. Bonadeo, I., Bottazzi, G & Lavazza, M. 'Echinacina B: polisaccaride attivo dell' echinacea." Riv. Ital. Essenze Profumi, 53, 281, 1971.
11. Chone, B. "Gezielte steuerung der leukozytentinetik durch echinacin." Arzneimittel-Forschung, 11, 611, 1965.
12. Buesing, K.H. "Inhibition of hyaluronidase by echinacin." Arzneimittel-Forschung, 2, 467-469, 1952.
13. Buesing, K.H. "Hyaluronidasehemmung als wirkungsmechanismus einiger therapeutisch nuzbarer naturstoffe." Arzneimittel-Forschung, 5(6), 320-322, 1955.
14. Koch, E. & Uebel, H. op. cit., 1953.
15. Kuhn, O. "Echinacea and phagocytosis." Arzneimittel-Forschung, 3, 194-200, 1953.
16. Tuennerhoff, F.K. & Schwabe, H.K. "Untersuchungen am menschen und am tier ueber den einfluss von echinacea-konzentraten auf die kuenstliche bindergewebsbildung nach fibrin-implantationen." Arzneimittel-Forschung, 6(6), 330-334, 1956.
17. Stimpel, M, Proksch, A., Wagner, H. & Lohmann-Matthes, M.L. "Macrophage activation and induction of macrophage cytotoxicity by purified polysaccharide fractions from the plant echinacea purpurea." Infection and Immunity, 46(3), 845-849, 1984.
18. Wagner, H., Riess-Maurer, J., Vollmar, A., Odenthal, S., Stuppner, H., Yurcic, K, Le Turdu, M. & Heur, H. "Immunstimulierend wirkende polysaccaride (Heteroglykane)

aus hoeheren pflanzen." Arzneimittel-Forschung, 34, 659-661, 1984.

19. Wagner, H. & Proksch, A. "Isolation of polysaccharides with immunostimulating activity from echinacea purpurea." International Conference Chem. Biotechnil. Biol. Act. Nat. Prod. (Proceedings), Atanasova, B. ed., 3(1), 200-202, 1981.

20. Wagner, H. & Proksch, A. "An immunostimulating active principle from echinacea purpurea." Zeitschrift fuer Agewandte Phytotherapie, 2(5), 166-168, 171, 1981.

21. Voaden, D.J. & Jacobson, M. "Tumor-inhibitors III. Identification and synthesis of an oncolytic hydrocarbon from american coneflower roots." Journal of Medicinal Chemistry, 15(6), 619-623, 1972.

22. Keller, H., inventor. "Recovery of active agents from aqueous extracts of the species of echinacea." Chemie Gruenenthal G.M.B.H., GER. 950,674, Oct 11, 1956.

23. Bonadeio, I., Bottazi, G. & Lavazza, M. "Echinacina B: polisaccaride attivo dell echinacea." Rev. Ital. Essenze Profumi, 53, 281, 1971.

24. Bonadeo, I. & Lavazza, M. "Echinacina B: suo azione sui fibroblasti." Riv Ital. Essenze Profumi, 54, 195, 1972.

25. Tragini, E., Tubaro, A., Melis, S. & Galli, L. "Evidence from two classic irritation tests for an anti-inflammatory action of a natural extract, echinacina B." Food and Chemical Toxicology, 23(2), 317-319, 1985.

26. Buesing, H.K. "Die beeinflussung des properdin-spiegels durch extrakte aus echinacea purpurea bei kaninchen." Zhurnal der immunitatsforschung, 115, 169-176, 1958.

27. Buesing, K.H. "The effect of extracts of echinacea purpurea on the properdin levels in rabbits." Zhurnal Immunitaetsforschung, 115, 169-176, 1958.

28. Wacker, A. & Hilbig, A. "Virus inhibition by echinacea purpurea." Planta Medica, 33, 89-102, 1978.

29. Wagner & Proksch, op. cit., 1981.

30. Quadripur, S.A. Therapie der Gegenwart, 115, 1072, 1976.

31. Reported in Foster, S. Echinacea Exalted!, Ozark Beneficial Plant Project, Missouri, 1985, p. 23.

32. Coeungniet, E. op. cit., 1986. 33. Lloyd, J.U. "Empiricism-Echinacea." Eclectic Medical Journal, 57(8), 421-427, 1897.

34. Felter, H.W. "Echinacea." Eclectic Medical Journal, 58, 79- 89, 1898.

35. Ellingwood, F. "Echinacea: the vegetable 'antitoxin', its characteristics and peculiar therapeutic effects." American Journal of Clinical Medicine, 21(11), 987-993, 1914.

36. Unruh, V. von. "Echinacea angustifolia and inula helenium in the treatment of tuberculosis." Nat. Eclec. Med. Assn. Qrt., Sept., 1915.

37. Liebstein, A.M. Eclectic Medical Journal, 1927, pp. 316-317, as quoted in Foster, S., op.cit.

38. Farnsworth, N. Hikino, A. & Wagner, H. Prog. Med. Econ. Pl. Res., Vol. 1, 1983, Academic Press.

39. Farnsworth, N.R. & Waller, D.P. "Current status of plant products reported to inhibit sperm." Research Frontiers in Fertility Regulation, 2(1), 1-16, 1982.

Ginkgo
(ginkgo biloba)

For The Brain And Nervous System

Guaranteed Potency Constituents.

Flavoglycosides (heterosides), and quercetin, as found in the leaf. These constituents should not be isolated, but should be present in a concentrated extract. Such an extract would be expected to contain about 24% flavoglycosides (about 10% of which should be quercetin and other naturally occurring flavonoids). The use of whole leaf is of little efficacy. The product is only effective when extracted and concentrated. In addition to the guaranteed potency constituents, a substantial amount of pharmacologically active terpene derivatives (ginkgolides and bilobalides) should also be present.

History.

The ginkgo biloba tree has been called "the doyen of trees," because of its antiquity.[1] It is believed to pre-date the ice age. Individual trees are believed capable of living 2000 to 4000 years, and some extant are dated to over a 1000 years. It is the sole remaining species of the so-called ginkgophyte botanical division which, according to fossil records, once flourished on the earth. Hence, ginkgo is also often called "a living fossil." The tree is basically native to China and Japan (though there is evidence it was native to Europe at some ancient date), but has been extensively cultivated throughout the world due to its hardy nature (even those of us with 'black thumbs' can grow a ginkgo.) Ginkgo biloba is remarkably resistant to all kinds of pollution, viruses and fungi. Possessed with a unique history, unique life cycle, and extremely unique biochemistry, is it any wonder it would be of unique and singular importance to man?

Asian cultures have used the **kernel** of ginkgo medicinally for hundreds of years. The body of folklore surrounding this practice is quite extensive. However, the modern Western use of ginkgo is limited exclusively to the **leaf**. A discussion of the folk medicine pertaining to the kernel would be meaningless in the context of this book,

63

and is therefore avoided. Since very little folk medicine has had a chance to develop concerning the leaf (the use of which begins seriously as recently as the early 1970's), the modern use of ginkgo is somewhat of an anomaly in herbal medicine, being almost completely without a body of historical experiential data upon which to build an experimental science. It is almost as if the modern scientific body of information on ginkgo sprang up overnight.

Ginkgo biloba extract is a complex product or compound, whose method of preparation has become very well-defined and exacting (there are, however, just a few labs in the world with the capability and know-how to do it). The green leaves of the tree are usually harvested from trees growing in plantations in South Korea, Japan and France. Growing, harvesting and extracting are perfectly standardized and controlled, insuring that all undesirable substances are eliminated and that certain levels of active constituents are obtained.[2]

There is one incidental point of interest. As will become clear in the following pages, ginkgo leaf extract holds enormous promise of extending the functional life of many people. Since the tree itself lives to such a ripe old age, is this (against all my protestations) in fact evidence for the validity of the Doctrine of Signatures?

Method of Action.

The presence of flavonoids in ginkgo biloba extract (Gbx) led early investigators to assume that Gbx would have some kind of action on the body's vascular system, since this is a major property of many flavonoids. Pharmacological tests in animals proved very encouraging, and subsequent clinical trials confirmed the action.

Cerebral vascular effects

In a typical pre-clinical study using standard pharmacological procedures, microscopic particles are injected into the carotid artery of rats to mimic arterial blockage. The administration of ginkgo biloba successfully protects the animals against the destructive effects of this procedure.[3] This particular experimental procedure has been carried out several times, always with the same results. And in some trials, additional interesting information has been obtained; namely, that under the influence of Gbx, increased levels of glucose and ATP occurred, which helped to maintain energy levels within individual cells.[4-6]

In the above procedures, following the injection of microspheres, there is usually a period of several hours characterized by a hypertensive burst, during which time considerable damage is done to the blood-brain barrier (that physiological system that prevents toxic substances from entering the brain mass from the surrounding blood vessels). The damage begins with just small molecules passing the barrier, but progresses until increasingly larger substances cross over. In later stages, considerable swelling (edema) of cerebral tissues becomes evident. The administration of Gbx during the initial stages prevents the later stages by stabilizing the membranes involved in the blood-brain barrier.[7] Other studies have shown that the stabilization takes place through *direct* action on the ionic potential across the membranes and *indirectly*, through action on intracellular (mitochondrial) respiration. These actions result in diminution of cerebral edema and essentially complete restoration of function.[8]

The term used to describe the physiological condition replicated in these studies is ischemia. This strange word simply refers to any decrease in blood flow, no matter what the cause. Arteriosclerosis is a kind of ischemia. Injecting microspheres into the carotid artery, or clamping it shut, are two experimental ways to produce cerebral ischemia or reduce the flow of blood to the brain. Whether produced experimentally, or through disease and degeneration, the results are the same. Edema is one of the major complications of cerebral ischemia. It is bad enough, itself, but, as indicated in preceding paragraphs, it is also an aggravating factor. It produces dramatic losses of intracellular energy and completely disrupts the delicate balance in concentrations of vital ions, both inside and outside of body cells, blood vessels and brain cells or neurons. In advanced stages, it involves the accumulation of lactic acid, inorganic phosphates, and free polyunsaturated fatty acids. Cerebral edema is one of the commonest complications of advancing age. It is profoundly important, then, that ginkgo biloba is able to inhibit the occurrence of cerebral edema and eliminate its neurological consequences.[9]

Platelet aggregation inhibition

In 1980, it was discovered that Gbx, like many other medicinal plants, had an inhibitory effect on blood platelet aggregation,[10] meaning that it effectively reduced the tendency of blood components to stick together; therefore, it reduced the tendency for dangerous clots or thrombi to form in veins and arteries. The ability to inhibit blood clotting implied, of course, that Gbx was probably an effective agent in the prevention of coronary thrombosis and in recovery from strokes and heart attacks, etc. The effect lasts for no more than a couple of hours after ingesting the ginkgo. This is good, because prolonged thinning of the blood could produce a dangerous tendency for excessive bleeding.

Free radical inhibition

One of the major effects of the cerebral vasogenic edema discussed above, is the production of arachidonic acid (a polyunsaturated fatty acid), which, in turn, is responsible for the formation of so-called membrane "aggressors," among which are found free radicals. In another line of basic research, Gbx demonstrated an ability to neutralize free radicals. That free radicals are directly implicated in the aging process as well as in many other debilitating conditions, is a reason why medical science is always in search of new and better ways to neutralize or destroy these pathological agents. Since oxygen is the major source of free radicals, oxygen scavengers are among the best substances used to prevent the formation of free radicals. The flavonoids of ginkgo, including quercetin, are extremely potent oxygen scavengers. Possessing a particular affinity for the central nervous system as well as the adrenal and thyroid glands, Gbx is ideally suited for use in protecting the heart, blood vessels, and brain against the destructive influence of free radicals.[11]

Free radical inhibition by Gbx has been reported in a number of petri dish models.[12] In this study, Gbx not only destroyed existing free radicals, but also inactivated their formation, and inhibited membrane lipid peroxidation (a destructive effect for which free radicals are partly responsible). Finally, through its anti-radical activity, Gbx exerted a stimulant effect on the biosynthesis of prostanoids (substances that, among other things, are capable of dilating blood vessels, thereby contributing to the prevention of high blood pressure).

One interesting animal model for the study of anti-radicals involves the simulation of diabetes in rats through the administration of alloxan; this procedure is regularly used for the investigation of substances hoped to be of value in the treatment of human diabetes. One of the side-effects of this procedure in rats (in exact replication of the same phenomenon in human diabetes) is the gradual impairment of visual function. It is now thought that this impairment is the result of the operation of free oxygenated radicals on the retina. Using this model, investigators have found that Gbx significantly prevents the onset and severity of visual impairment, probably because of its effect on free radicals.[13]

In other experimental models involving the visual apparatus, ginkgo has likewise demonstrated anti-radical properties. For example, one team of researchers found that Gbx significantly improved long distance visual acuity in human patients suffering from senile macular degeneration (a troublesome opacity of the pupils, that occurs in the elderly). Free oxygenated radicals are thought to be the cause of this condition.[14] It should be noted that macular degeneration is a condition for which there is no satisfactory medical treatment. Recent findings that oxygenated free radicals are formed under the action of sunlight suggests the usefulness of oxygen scavengers in treatment. The effectiveness of Gbx supports this theory. Finally, Gbx displays protection against laser-induced lesions of retinal cells. Such lesions are related to the production of free radicals in a fairly complex manner. The investigators concluded that pretreatment with Gbx, by capturing the free radicals, prevented significant tissue damage.[15]

Neurotransmitters (Nervous system communication)

We next encounter a series of studies that impact on the health of the nervous system and those vascular and endocrine systems that both support it and depend on it for their own health. Originally, rat studies were carried out in which the carotid artery was tied off to reduce blood flow to the brain. It was found that pretreatment with Gbx significantly increased blood flow, an important finding itself — but, perhaps more critical to the present discussion, it also produced a significant rise in *dopamine* synthesis.[16] Dopamine is a *neurotransmitter*, or a substance critical to the transfer of information among nerves, and between nerves and structures of the body such as muscles, glands, organs, and blood vessels. The remarkable adaptablity of the body and mind rests upon this principle. The structures that carry information throughout the body are not 'hard-wired.' Rather, there are numerous 'junctions' or synapses, where nerves terminate and originate. Electrical impulses traveling along nerves are transmitted across these gaps chemically, thereby allowing the impulse along one nerve to be transmitted to several neurons at the junction. If one neuron can affect ten others, then those ten can get even more neurons involved at the next junction, and so forth. There are even gaps between nerves and the group of muscle or gland cells at which they terminate. Neurotransmitters are the chemicals released in the gaps by neural impulses. Without them all activity — neural, muscular, glandular, everything — would cease. Many common poisons, such as strychnine and morphine, directly affect the concentration, composition and effectiveness of neurotransmitters (in fact, the list of toxic plant substances that operate in this manner is long indeed — and includes substances such as atropine and scopolamine found in common cold remedies). Substances that beneficially affect transmitters have great implications for health, the quality of life, and even the prospect of longevity. Thus, the finding that Gbx increased the level of dopamine provided a powerful stimulus for further research on the effects of Gbx on aging and mental functioning in general. And dopamine was not destined to be the only neurotransmitter discovered that was affected by Gbx.

Further evidence for the involvement of dopamine came from the study of the effects of Gbx on the isolated intestine of the guinea pig. It was already known that Gbx inhibited the action of histamine-induced contractions of this organ,[17] but subsequent study was able to tease apart the mechanism of action still further, only to discover that the action of Gbx involved dopaminergic and histaminergic receptors (sites on the muscle that do not respond to neural stimulation without the presence of either dopamine or histamine).[18]

Studies on the contractile action of Gbx on isolated rabbit aorta found that this action was probably due to the ability of substances to stimulate the release of still other neurotransmitters: the *catecholamines*, namely *epinephrine* and *norepinephrine*.[19] Because of its capacity to release catecholamines, Gbx could affect the functioning of the entire network of catecholaminergic glandular, cardiovascular and nervous systems of the body (perhaps the most extensive network upon which depends the most important functions of life). This line of reasoning led researchers to continue the search for Gbx's effects on neurotransmitters. Studies confirmed and extended the original findings to include effects on virtually the entire chemical basis for nervous system and cardiovascular functioning.[20-22]

One study of particular importance found that Gbx exerts a specific effect on the *noradrenergic* system (noradrenergic is the name of the nervous system that depends primarily on the presence of norepinephrine), as well as on *beta-receptors*.[23] Beta receptor sites, when activated, produce among other things dilation of airways in the lung, and dilation of peripheral blood vessels — i.e, those going to muscles, etc. The best description of the effect of Gbx on the noradrenergic system is that of 'reactivation.' In the aging process, this system, especially in the brain, begins to lose vigor; associated symptoms of memory loss, speech defects, and decrease in alertness appear. By reactivating the noradrenergic system of the cerebral cortex, Gbx promises to be an important substance in the prevention of premature aging.

Note: The mechanism of action of Gbx on the isolated rabbit aorta is very complex (even when not considering the differential effects of the many constituents in Gbx), involving the release of stored norepinephrine by tyramine which is itself a precursor in the synthesis of all catecholamines, and the stimulation and inhibition of neurotransmission by a myriad other chemicals present at the synapse. After scientists have had sufficient opportunity to unravel these complex interactions, perhaps we will learn more about the precise manner in which Gbx is able to achieve some of its more dramatic therapeutic effects (as in cerebrovascular insufficiency and peripheral vascular disorders). Ultimately, I suspect, we will see that Gbx, in keeping with the action of many of the most beneficial herbal products, is tonic in nature, and acts by restoring healthy function, no matter which way it departs from normal.

Whereas the adrenergic and noradrenergic division of the nervous system underlies behavior that can best be characterized by the *increased use* of energy (extreme examples would be flight and fight), there is another division responsible for energy *conservation* and storage. The *cholinergic* system is just as important to survival and quality of life as the adrenergic. But different neurotransmitters (acetylcholine, for instance) and receptor sites are involved. A decline in function of this system is also implicated in the aging process and the onset of dementia. Using the rat as a model of this condition, researchers have found that the oral administration of Gbx significantly increases the population of appropriate cholinergic receptor sites in the brain.[24] So, rather than having a direct effect on transmitter substances, in this case the compound works by proliferating sites that can be activated by cholinergic neurotransmitters. That end result is the same: revitalization of decreasingly effective cerebral tissue.

In looking for the mechanism of action of Gbx on the nervous system, researchers[25] have discovered the following factors:

* A direct action on both arteries and veins to increase blood flow to the brain;

* Stimulation of neurotransmitter release into the synapse;

* Inhibition of enzymatic breakdown of neurotransmitters (if just a little neurotransmitter is being produced you don't want it to be destroyed too soon — in healthy systems you wouldn't want to interfere with normal enzymatic function);

* Stimulation of the release of endogenous relaxing factors in the arterial endothelium (such as prostacyclin and EDRF).

Conclusion

If the basic research discussed above seems trivial, boring and inconsequential, its implications for human health and its impact on subsequent clinical research is of a most profound nature. Research normally builds upon itself, like a brick building, layer upon layer. The foundation is almost always formed of a mass of seemingly incoherent bits and pieces which, nonetheless, come together to form a solid body of data upon which the life protecting and enhancing structures are ultimately built. In this case, the individual indications of the involvement of neurotransmitters, oxygen scavengers, platelet ag-gregation inhibitors, vascularity and so forth has led rapidly to theories involving the entire cardiovascular and nervous systems.

Therapeutic Research.

From the basic experimental trials reviewed above, research jumped quickly to the human arena. This was possible because of the large body of information already available on flavonoids in general, especially on two of the major flavonoids in ginkgo: quercetin and kampferol. It was originally thought that much the same effects would be seen with ginkgo as were obtained from other flavonoids. For the most part, that was true, but some surprises were in store.

Vascular Effects

In one of the earliest screening trials in humans using ginkgo biloba extract, some important results of pre-clinical trials were con-firmed: Gbx exerts considerable anti-spasmodic or sedative effects, and has excellent restorative effects on the nervous system.[26] In one study, over one hundred patients with organic and neurological angiopathy (angiopathy refers to any disease of the vessels) as well as ten healthy volunteers were observed for changes in several physiological parameters resulting from exercise after using Gbx. It was concluded that Gbx treatment should be considered in any case of central and peripheral vascular disease. Interestingly, it was also found that Gbx should be an effective treatment for diabetic angiopathy as it decreases the consumption of insulin.

In persons recovering from thrombosis (blood clot in artery of heart) it was found that Gbx lowered blood pressure and dilated peripheral blood vessels, including the capillaries.[27]

One of the problems in the use of normal vasodilators is that of lack of constancy in action. The ensuing unpredictability in their use can present complications with dire consequences for the patient. In trials comparing ginkgo to other vasodilators, it has been found that ginkgo extract is significantly more constant in its action, and is there-fore a more reliable agent.[28]

In efforts to tease apart the effects of Gbx on circulation, inves-tigators have looked at the manner in which the extract affects the microcirculation of the conjunctiva in elderly patients suffering from disturbances in cerebral blood supply. These studies have found a consistent increase in capillary and venous blood flow to the head resulting from decreased resistance to flow. This increase in flow was not accompanied by hypotension or any appreciable variations in blood pressure.[29-30]

Some observers view the action of Gbx on venous tone as regulatory rather than as a simple increase, since the herbal extract corrects venular spasms that often occur in elderly, often arteriosclerotic, patients. The regulatory action makes ginkgo a unique product — at one and the same time able to combat disturbances resulting from vascular spasm, and able, with the same efficiency, to restore tone and circulation in areas subject to vasomotor paralysis.[31] In a similar vein (no pun intended), it has been found that the use of Gbx avoids another common complication caused by the more orthodox hypotensive medications: it increases peripheral blood flow without sacrificing cerebral circulation. A common side-effect of standard peripheral vaso-dilators is that blood tends to accumulate in the peripheral vessels rather than circulate to the vessels of the central nervous system, whose supporting vascular micro-structure is not affected by the drug. Gbx avoids this complication by simultaneously increasing blood flow to the periphery and to the brain.

With 20 patients between the ages of 62 and 86 years serving as subjects, a 1977 study attempted to discover the effect of very low doses of Gbx, administered over a two week period. All subjects were diagnosed as experiencing a lack of adequate blood supply to the brain (cerebral circulatory insufficiency) due to age and arteriosclerosis. The expectation of the investigators was that the combination of age, health of subjects, and the low dosage, would preclude any kind of spectacular results. Yet, of 20 subjects, 15 responded dramatically with much improved cerebral hemodynamics.[32]

In is not surprising, then, that in a recent six month long study in patients with peripheral arterial insufficiency, Gbx was able to produce significant improvement in all experimental measures, including measures of ability to walk long distances without pain, and on the blood flow to the legs. The experimenters describe the results as not only statistically significant, but as clinically remarkable.[33]

Administered to patients with Parkinson's disease secondary to cerebral arteriosclerosis, Gbx increased blood supply to the brain and improved its nutritional status. The latter finding has not been investigated thoroughly. But it crops up now and again usually as a by-product of a study rather than as the subject proper of the study.[34]

Instead of presenting a detailed analysis of every study on vascularity, I will briefly review the most important, as follows (over 95% of the following studies were double-blind placebo controlled trials):

* 65% successful treatment of 30 patients with focal or diffuse cerebral vascular disease.[35]

71

* 80% successful treatment of 47 patients with cerebral circulatory insufficiency, measured as improvement in mental functioning, EEG parameters, and cerebral angiogram. This study was a good demonstration of the potential benefit of Gbx in the treatment of disease with both neuro and circulatory components.[36]

* 80% success rate in 60 patients with chronic cerebral insufficiency as measured by improvement in functional symptoms, such as vertigo, headache, etc.[37]

* successful treatment of 60 patients with cerebral insufficiency, as measured by ECG, EEG, computer tomography of the skull, and psychological tests.[38]

* 92% success rate in patients with cerebrovascular insufficiency in which all pathological findings disappeared after 18 days of treatment.[39]

* 80% success in treating headache and lesser per cent success in case of migraine, though still highly significant considering subjects had complained of migraine for a long time and had already received other treatments — authors concluded that Gbx should be considered as one of the most effective treatments for migraine.[40]

* 23 of 30 cases of dystrophy that follows venous insufficiency and is a complication of varicose disease or postphlebitic disease — successfully treated.[41]

* 40% success in the treatment of 49 elderly patients with peripheral arteriopathy (arterial insufficiency of lower limbs), some with angiopathy complicating senile diabetes mellitus, as measured by improvement in general psychophysical performance and in capacity to adapt to the environment.[42]

* 72% success in the treatment of chronic vasculopathies that are normally treated with vasodilators, which, unfortunately, end by lowering vascular tone, rather than restoring it; Gbx acts by toning the arterioles to produce the vasodilator effect.[43]

* 82% success in a study similar to one above, as measured by maximum walking distance, oscillometric index, mean blood pressure, plethysmography and systolic blood pressure.[44]

* successful treatment of 21 patients with the very severe and rapidly disabling vascular disease of the lower limbs called chronic arterial obliteration, as measured both instrumentally and functionally; recommendation made that Gbx be used for all patients with this disease unless surgery was impending.[45]

* significant reduction of pain in patients with obstructive arteriopathy.[46]

Vascular disturbances of the inner ear

Both structural and functional disturbances of the inner ear have been successfully treated with Gbx These problems all stem from some underlying vascular defect. In one study Gbx was given to persons suffering from hearing loss due to old age (presbyacusia), patients with persistent ringing in the ears, and patients with vertigo. Improved hearing was experienced by 40% of the presbyacusia patients; those who didn't respond were assumed to have irreversible lesions of the sensory structures of the inner ear. Most of those patients with ringing in the ear experienced significant improvement within 10-20 days. The action of Gbx on cerebral circulation resulted in swift and complete disappearance of vertigo. The researcher concluded his study with the admonition to use Gbx, not only for treatment, but for prevention of otorhinolaryngeal problems.[47]

Similar results were obtained by various other investigators.[48-50] An 88% success rate was obtained in one study involving 49 patients suffering variously from hearing loss, ringing, vertigo and labyrinthine syndrome.[35] The consensus of such studies is that Gbx is highly effective in neurosensory diseases of the inner ear of vascular origin which manifest themselves by ringing in the ear, vertigo and headache.

That severe cochleovestibular disturbances, with a vascular component, are subject to amelioration by Gbx, is reported in a recent study. In deafness of long standing, the results were poor, but even then definite improvement was seen in about half of the cases. Such results are truly remarkable. In recent deafness, following head injuries or sonic damage, the results were very good in more than 60% of the cases. Ringing in the ear improved significantly, even in very severe cases, at a rate of 74%. Almost all patients with vertigo reported significant improvement.[37]

In one study, devoted explicitly to vertigo, 70 patients were given Gbx or placebo over a 3 month period. The effectiveness of the Gbx on the intensity, frequency and duration of the disorder was statistically significant. At the end of the trial, 47% of the patients receiving Gbx were completely free of their symptoms (18% of the placebo group recovered).[51] Other studies have essentially replicated the findings of this one.[52-54]

Proctology

Patients suffering from acute and chronic hemorrhoids have benefited from the use of Gbx. One early study reported good, or very good, results in 86% of several dozen patients with conditions such as

73

hemorrhoids in a more or less advanced stage. The compound was particularly effective in individuals with congestive conditions and bleeding.[55] Gbx appears to have less effect on fissures, but is very good at relieving pain and stopping rectal bleeding.[56-57]

Mental and behavioral effects

It should be realized that, in order for changes in behavior to occur, fundamental changes in the underlying blood supply to the brain and in the status of neurotransmission must first occur. This concept may seem too mechanistic for some, but the data clearly indicate that overt behavior, whether it be sensory-related (reading) or purely cognitive (thinking rationally), depends upon an healthy nervous system. The studies to be reviewed in this section reflect gross measurements for which internal changes are mostly assumed. In a way, these studies are the final verification of the value of all the other work on vascularity, neural transmission, edema and so forth.

In a recent 12 week study, elderly patients expressing no particular complaint were selected to receive Gbx(120mg) or placebo on a daily basis. EEG readings were taken daily, and certain behavioral and psychometric tasks were engaged in. Gbx produced definite improvements in alertness measures in persons in whom there was room for improvement, but induced no change in the persons whose initial performance was already at a high level.[58] In comparison to controls, the experimental subjects showed a substantial increase in vigilance, as measured by simple reaction time tests and multiple choice reaction tests. These results contrasted somewhat with results obtained in an earlier trial, in which healthy young girls improved significantly on a memory test, after ingesting 600 mg of Gbx.[59] The general implication of these studies is that Gbx increases the rate of information processing at neuronal levels, not only in geriatric persons with deteriorating mental function, but perhaps also in healthy young individuals.

In a more recent research effort, eight healthy female volunteers were administered variable doses of Gbx, one hour before being subjected to a battery of tests, including critical flicker fusion (when do two flickers look like one), choice reaction time, subjective rating scale, and the Sternberg memory scanning test (a measure of short term memory). A 600 mg dose produced significant differences in scores on the Sternberg test; the first three measures were not affected. These results differentiate Gbx from sedative and stimulant drugs (which would affect the first three tests) and suggest a selective effect of Gbx on the memory process.[60] Note that these tests took place just one hour following the administration of the compound. This immediate effect, when compared to the longer periods required for the vascular action, suggest a wide range of properties attributable to this herb.

Utilizing the full power of the EEG, one study determined the effects of Gbx in three pathological animal models, in young healthy volunteers and in elderly people with dementia disorders. It was found that the EEG tracings correlated well with the psychometric tests employed. The results confirmed those of other clinical trials and especially highlighted the ability of Gbx to enhance alertness in the human subjects.[61]

Not many long term studies have had a chance to be conducted, given the short history of ginkgo research, but one such study was recently reported. Using 166 patients, researchers tracked the effects of Gbx on a battery of behavioral, clinical and physiological measures (such as those discussed elsewhere) of cerebral disorders due to aging. Differences between control and treatment groups became clearly apparent after just three months. Over the ensuing months, the differences increased — a dramatic demonstration of benefits available from the use of ginkgo extract.[62]

Alzheimer's disease

Everything that has been said so far in this chapter points to the potential use of Gbx in one disease that has consistently avoided adequate treatment and cure: Alzheimer's disease. Alzheimer's is one of those conditions that is still ill-defined in the literature, has an even more vague etiology, and necessarily resists therapeutic interventions and prognostications. There are not even any established objective evaluation scales that allow the observer the means for accurately and unambiguously determining the occurrence or extent of improvement following medication.

Essentially, what we have are subjective evaluations, based mostly on subjects' self-reports of their overall well-being; semi-objective measures are, currently, extremely limited. In people between the ages of 50 and 65, in whom well-established symptoms of advanced senile dementia are not yet present, but who appear to be experiencing recurrent bouts of forgetfulness, incoordination, failing speech, visual and auditory problems and so forth, Gbx produces periods of decreased intensity and duration, as well as lowered measures of frequency for any given manifestation.

A review of the research on *causes* of Alzheimer's produces some terms we have used already in this chapter: free radical damage, vascular insufficiency, ischemia, cholinergic and noradrenergic dysfunction. A review of *symptoms* of Alzheimer's likewise produces a familiar list: loss of memory and mental acuity, visual impairment, auditory loss, cerebral edema, varices, thrombosis, spasms, and so forth. Again, *clinically*, we have seen that Gbx has proved active on circulatory and rheological functions, on neuronal and metabolic consequences of ischemia and hypoxia, on neurotransmission, and on membrane resistance to free radical damage.[63] It is hard to resist the hypothesis that Gbx could be an invaluable aid in the treatment and prevention of Alzheimer's disease.

Research along these lines is currently underway, and preliminary discussions are extremely promising.[64-65] Patients are significantly improving in walking ability, treadmill performance, visual acuity, hearing, equilibrium, mood and other subjective measures, and in electro-encephlographic (EEG) measures.

In reviewing the available research, one scientist concluded that ginkgo extract showed exceptional promise as the drug of choice "in all types of dementia, and even in patients suffering from cognitive disorders secondary to depression, because of its beneficial effects on mood. Of special concern are people who are just beginning to experience deterioration in their cognitive function. Ginkgo biloba extract might delay deterioration and enable these subjects to maintain a normal life and escape institutionalization. In addition, Gbx appears to be a safe substance, being well tolerated, even in doses many times higher than those usually recommended.[66] We can only concur with this statement.

Therapeutic Use.

Because of its pharmacological properties, Gbx is now widely used in Europe for treating many forms of vascular diseases. But, it has not yet been introduced to the United States by the pharmaceutical industry. This has left the door open to distribution by American--based botanical companies. Gbx can be found in most health food stores.

A survey of packaging information on European products produces an impressive list of uses and recommendations for Ginkgo preparations: vertigo; headache; tinnitus; inner ear disturbances including partial deafness; impairment of memory and ability to concentrate; diminished intellectual capacity and alertness as a result of insufficient circulation to the brain; anxiety, depression, neurological disorders; complications of stroke and skull injuries; diminished sight and hearing ability due to vascular insufficiency; cramp-like pains in the calf muscle while walking and intermittent claudication as a result of arterial obstruction; a feeling of deafness, a sensitivity to cold and pallor in the toes due to peripheral circulatory insufficiency; the more severe Raynaud's disease, a vasospastic disorder characterized by pallor and cyanosis of the fingers with or without gangrene; hormonal and neural based disorders as well as angiopathic trophic disorders; arterial circulatory disturbances due to aging, diabetes and nicotine abuse; cerebral vascular and nutritional insufficiency; sclerosis of cerebral arteries with and without mental manifestations; arteriosclerotic angiopathy of lower limbs; diabetic tissue damage with danger of gangrene; chronic arterial obliteration; circulatory disorders of skin tissues as well as skin ulcerations caused by insufficient supplies of blood, oxygen and nourishment; cellular metabolic disturbances.

Vascular insufficiency

The primary therapeutic property of ginkgo is to increase the flow of blood into areas previously deprived of this life-giving substance to one degree or another, including the brain, the lower limbs, all arteries, veins, even the smallest capillaries. Upon this principle depend almost all other properties. We devoted considerable space to the presentation of the basic and clinical research validating the vascular effects of Gbx. Scientists have devoted considerable time and effort in trying to understand those effects. First, in basic or pre-clinical settings researchers evolved several models of vascular insufficiency. Their primary question was, "How many different ways can we restrict the flow of blood to critical parts of the body; and how well will Gbx prevent, reduce or inhibit damaging consequences?" As we saw, Gbx passed the tests with flying colors. In virtually no instance was the compound ineffective, and in many cases its effectiveness was astounding.

Second, we saw how doctors and medical scientists applied the ginkgo extract in clinical settings, using real live patients as subjects. The main question was, "How many different kinds and manifestations of vascular insufficiency (ischemia) will respond to Gbx?" And a related question, "How do healthy volunteers respond?" Again, the answers to these questions were extremely encouraging. Whether vascular insufficiency was arterial or venous, peripheral or central, functional or structural — it didn't matter — Gbx was significantly effective in the vast majority of cases. One salient finding was that it took more Gbx to produce a noticeable effect in healthy volunteers than it took to produce a significant improvement in the health of patients suffering from acute or chronic insufficiency. The universal opinion of scientists is that the earlier treatment begins, the better the chances for complete recovery, especially from the more serious as Alzheimer's. But even in advanced cases, improvement begins almost immediately and continues over a period of many months. The total extent of possible improvement is undetermined at this time, because the substance has not been in use long enough to determine an end point.

It is sometimes difficult to give names to the various conditions that arise as a result of ischemia. Almost every cell of the body will suffer when there is an inadequate supply of blood. The whole body deteriorates. One suffers from lack of energy, susceptibility to infection, decreased mental and physical function, and so forth. Dementia in the elderly is primarily a problem of inadequate circulation, but it can take one of several different forms, depending on a host of other factors. So, as we review the effects of Gbx on the underlying vascular and cellular manifestations of disease, it will often be up to the reader to draw his own conclusions, to recognize the signs in himself or his acquaintances. Various constellations of symptoms are possible, and not all combinations have names. Here, then is my own summary of findings and their implications.

Gbx has been shown to be involved in health and disease in the following ways.

* by directly contributing to the metabolic health of cells (anabolic and eutrophic); by increasing levels of glucose and ATP; by helping to maintain energy levels.

* by stabilizing ionic potentials across membranes; by stabilizing the blood brain barrier, thereby preventing or reducing cerebral edema and hypertension; by stimulating mitochondrial respiration; by preventing and curing headaches and migraines.

* by retarding the onset of dementia that results from sclerosis of cerebral arteries; by reducing the effects of progressive cerebral circulatory insufficiency due to age; by increasing overall health of cerebral tissue.

* by sedative and antispasmodic effects on the nervous system.

* by decreasing the consumption of insulin and thereby being of potential use in cases of diabetic angiopathy; by having practically no affect on glucose metabolism, and thereby being especially well-suited for use by diabetics, who generally suffer greatly from insufficient circulation.

* by lowering blood pressure and dilating peripheral blood vessels, and thereby serving as a treatment for hypertension and as an aid in persons recovering from coronary thrombosis.

* by being a more reliable agent compared to others; by regulating vascular properties, rather than just increasing them; by stabilizing activity; by being a 'tonic' and not just a simple drug, and thereby

being equally good for treating vascular spasms and for restoring tone following vasomotor paralysis; by demonstrating a consistent super-iority to other vasodilators and hypotensive agents.

* by reversing the effects of peripheral arterial insufficiency; by increasing the ability to walk without pain (and hence being a good treatment for intermittent claudication).

* by treating both the circulatory and neurological components of disease.

* by demonstrating effectiveness over a wide range of symp-toms, from the simple, such as varicose veins, to the complex and dan-gerous, such as chronic arterial obliteration.

Finally, it must be said that we are still in the first stages of research on the vascular properties of Gbx. There is still much to be learned about the intricate interactions among the body's cardio-vascular, endocrine and nervous systems and about the therapeutic manner in which Gbx intervenes. Much more awaits to be found, explicated and applied in a meaningful way.

Platelet Aggregation Inhibition

Closely related to vascular effects, but usually treated separately, is the ability to inhibit the tendency of blood cells (platelets) to stick to-gether like old pancakes. Like other agents in this class, we can expect Gbx to effectively protect the arteries and veins of the body against the formation of dangerous blood clots or thrombi.

Free Radical Inhibition

Research on the effects of free radicals on the human body is also still in its infancy, but theoretical and empirical data suggest that free radicals are inherently involved in the aging process and in degener-ative diseases such as cancer, diabetes, blindness, atherosclerosis and so forth. Free radicals are generated by the natural metabolic processes of the body. Obviously, there is no way to prevent aging; and it may be that free radicals are ultimately the cause of natural death. And everybody dies. So we are not looking for a way to completely remove the presence of free radicals or their effects from the body. The consequences of such an effort would probably be far worse than the effects of the free radicals themselves.

Rather, our goal is to keep free radical formation from running amok. Unfortunately, we live in an age in which there are increasingly more environmental sources of free radicals and causes for free radical formation — from the foods we eat to the air we breath, to the water we drink. The oxygen atom and oxygen-containing molecules are intrinsically involved in the formation of free radicals. Although it is necessary for life, the oxygen atom may also be responsible for death. In the biblical periods, during which people lived to be hundreds of years old, perhaps the world was a little freer of environmental sources of free radicals. At any rate, in today's world, the body is forced to work overtime in producing substances (enzymes) such as S.O.D. and G.T.P. (superoxide dismutase and glutathione peroxidase) which neutralize these free radicals.

In recent years, health-minded individuals have tried to augment the body's own anti-radical processes by supplementing the diet with S.O.D. and other substances (beta-carotene, selenium, Vitamins C & E, etc.) In my view, nutritional supplements simply augment the effects of the oxygen scavengers from the plant kingdom. In many experimental trials, Gbx has shown considerable ability to act as an oxygen scavenger and directly prevent the occurrence of free radical damage. The presence of very potent flavonoids in the ginkgo biloba extract is primarily responsible for plant's high degree of anti-oxidant activity. Plant flavonoids as a group possess anti-oxidant activity, but some, such as those found in ginkgo, milk thistle and centella, appear to be more active than others. What is more remarkable is the apparent ability of certain kinds of flavonoids to concentrate in certain specific areas of the body; our state of knowledge on the properties of flavonoids is not advanced far enough yet to explain this phenomenon, but it does appear to be a valid effect: ginkgo flavonoids concentrate in certain glands and in the nervous system, especially in the area of synapses between nerves and blood vessels (but other receptor sites also appear to be involved).

Inner ear problems

Inner ear problems represent an interesting sub-class of problems involving insufficient eutrophic support from the vascular system. Any problem of the inner ear that has resulted from a disturbance in blood supply (and most such problems have a vascular component) can be beneficially affected by the ingestion of Gbx.

* Vertigo. The research indicates that over half of the people suffering from acute and chronic vertigo can expect total recovery from this problem if they ingest Gbx daily for several weeks. The exact dose is difficult to ascertain, but the minimal amounts suggested later in this chapter should be sufficient. It does little good to use more, since the body can only utilize so much at a time. Excess is simply eliminated.

* Tinnitus or ringing in the ears. This is another condition that

usually has a vascular component. Most clinical cases recover completely after using Gbx.

   * Hearing loss. Studies have been promising for certain kinds of hearing loss. The outlook is best if deafness is the result of head injuries, sonic damage or vascular problems of recent origin. In cases where hearing loss or partial deafness has been present for a long time, the prognosis is not as good, but, even here, about half of the people treated have experienced definite improvement.

Proctology

   Just a brief note is required here. Many proctological problems are also the result of aberrant vascularity. Therefore, one would expect Gbx to be of some value. And indeed it is. The chronic hemorrhoid sufferer can expect immediate and sustained improvement while using the ginkgo extract. Studies have recorded significant improvement in congestion, bleeding, and pain in over 80% of the patients observed.

Effects on neurophysiology

   As indicated in the preceding paragraph, Gbx seems to have a natural affinity for the nervous system. It also seems to concentrate in the vascular and endocrine systems that strongly affect the function of the nervous system. Chief among these is the adrenal gland that is responsible for producing dopamine, epinephrine and norepinephrine as well as intermediary products required in the formation, activity and metabolism of other neurotransmitters. Gbx is also, through its affects on blood flow, able to improve the availability of still another critically important neurotransmitter: acetylcholine. This is the neurotransmitter that is affected by lecithin ingestion. Unlike Gbx, lecithin does not affect all of the other neurotransmitters.

   Gbx effects the nervous system in the following ways:

   * by concentrating in the adrenal gland; by stimulating the synthesis of important neurotransmitters, and thereby increasing the capacity for normal physical activity, including voluntary behavior as well as involuntary, vegetative functions such as digestion, rejuvenation, blood pressure regulation, hormone secretion, blood sugar regulation, and so forth.

   * by increasing the flow of blood to the brain thereby stimulating the growth of receptor sites, which leads ultimately to increased cerebral capacity, which is, in turn, manifested by improved memory and reasoning power, improved mood, improved reaction time, alertness, speech and so forth.

* by directly inhibiting the breakdown of neurotransmitters in the synapse; by increasing the time such neurotransmitters are available during any given period of neural stimulation, thereby helping to insure that critical information is processed efficiently by the nervous system, especially in life-threatening situations; thereby also contributing to quality of life as evidenced by improvement in mood, memory and self- mastery.

* by stimulating the release of neurotransmitters into the synapse (neurotransmitters are normally present in small 'sacks' or vesicles in the ends of the neuron 'sending the message' and are released into the synapses in response to a message arriving at the synapse); by contributing in this fashion still another increment in the improvement of all life functions that depend upon the nervous system.

Mental and behavioral manifestations

Happily, all of the clinical studies conducted to date confirm that the many underlying vascular, endocrine and neuronal effects of Gbx surface in a manifold way as influences on observable behavior, sense of well- being, decreased hospitalization, capacity for self-sufficiency and similar measures.

High doses of Gbx even improve short term mental processes in healthy volunteers, a remarkable finding that may shape the manner in which college students cram for exams.

But the real potential for Gbx lies in its possible benefits for delaying the onset of dementia and for reversing the course of this dreaded condition. Virtually anybody, whether they are already experiencing the effects of aging on mental function, or just approaching that point, can benefit from the use of Gbx. The middle-aged can postpone the onset of mental and behavioral deterioration, or perhaps even avoid it altogether; the aged can regain some substantial degree of mental vigor and reverse the downward spiral of mental senility.

Many more studies need to be undertaken before we will know with any exactitude just how much improvement is possible, in memory restoration, in alertness, in learning potential, and finally, in the avoidance and treatment of the whole Alzheimer's disease syndrome.

Route of Administration.

The standard way of using Gbx is orally. Injections are sometimes used, but all important therapeutic effects are observed following the simple ingestion of tablet or capsule.

Dosage.

It takes time to rebuild veins and nerves. Use small amounts for long periods for best results. You can find Gbx in varying dosages. I suggest you look for a guarantee of potency on the label, since this is by far the best. Generally, the potency can be expressed in a couple of ways, either as the amount of Gbx or as the amount of flavoglycosides (heterosides) present. Ideally, both numbers will be indicated. Since quercetin is one of the most important flavoglycosides, its concentration could also be indicated; if it isn't, chances are no special effort was made during production to insure that a certain level of quercetin is present.

The more advanced production methods are now able to concentrate higher amounts of flavoglycosides in smaller amounts of extract. A larger capsule does not necessarily mean a greater activity. In fact, the most advanced product to date can be found in the smallest capsule with greatest concentration of active principles: a 60 mg capsule with 14.4 mg (24%) of flavoglycosides (of which 6 mg, or 10% should be quercetin and other flavonoids). That's potent. Take two a day.

Toxicity.

Before Gbx was ever approved for human consumption it had been extensively tested for potential side effects. Virtually none were found. Some people have reported mild gastrointestinal upset, headache or skin rash that are probably allergic in nature, but that's it. Even doses many times in excess of the recommended therapeutic amount have not produced significant toxicity.

One long term study was carried out to determine if very large doses of Gbx had any influence on delicate endocrine balances. The results of all hormonal and blood assays were negative.[67]

References.

1. Michel, P.F. "Le doyen des arbres: le ginkgo biloba." Presse Med., 15(31), 1450-4, 1986.
2. Drieu, K. "Preparation et definition de l'extrait de ginkgo biloba." Presse Med., 15(31), 1455-7, 1986.
3. Larsen, R.G., Dupeyron, J.P., Boulu, R.G., "Modele d'eschemie cerebrale experimentale par microspheres chez le rat. Etude de l'effect de deux extraits de ginkgo biloba et du naftidrofuril." Therapie, 33, 651, 1978.
4. Rapin, J.R. & Le Poncin-Lafitte, M. "Modele experimental d'ischemie cerebrale. Action preventive de l'extrait de ginkgo." Sem. Hop. Paris, 55, 2047, 1979.
5. Le Poncin-Lafitte, M., Rapin, J., Rapin J.R. "Effects of ginkgo biloba on changes induced by quantitative cerebral microembolization in rats." Arch. Int. Pharmacodyn., 243, 236, 1980.

6. Rapin, J.R. & Le Poncin-Lafitte, M. "Consommation cerebrale du glucose. Effet de l'extrait de ginkgo biloba." Presse Med., 15(31), 1494-7, 1986.
7. Grosdemouge, C, Le Poncin-Lafitte, & Rapin, J.R. "Effets protecteurs de l'extrait de ginkgo biloba sure la rupture precoce de la barriere hemoencephalique le rat." Presse Med., 15(31), 1502-1505, 1986.
8. Spinnewyn, B., Blavet, N. & Clostre, F. "Effets de l'extrait de ginkgo biloba sure un modele d'ischemie cerebrale chez la gerbille." Presse Med., 15(31), 1511-1986.
9. Etienne, A., Hecquet, F. & Clostre, F. "Mecanismes d'action de l'extrait de ginkgo biloba sure l'oedeme cerebral experimental." Presse Med., 15(31), 1506-1510, 1986.
10. Borzeix, M.G., Labos, M. & Hartl, C. "Recherches sure l'action antiagregant de l'extrait de ginkgo biloba. Activite au niveau des arteres et des veines de la pie-mere chez le lapin." Arch. Int. Pharmacodyn., 243, 236, 1980.
11. Brunello, N., Racagni, G., Clostre, F., Drieu, K., & Braquet, P., "Effects of an extract of ginkgo biloba on noradrenergic systems of rat cerebral cortex." Pharm. Res. Commun., 17, 1063-72, 1985. 12. Pincemail, J. & Deby, C. "Proprietes antiradicalaires de l'extrait de ginkgo biloba." Presse Med., 15(31), 1475-9, 1986.
13. Doly, M., Droy-Lefaix, M.T., Bonhomme, B. & Braquet, P. "Effet de l'extrait de ginkgo biloba sur l'electrophysiologie de la retine isolee de rat diabetique." Presse Med., 15(31), 1480- 3, 1986.
14. Lebuissen, D.A., Leroy, L. & Rigal, G. "Traitement des degenerescences 'maculaires seniles' par l'extrait de ginkgo biloba. Etude preliminaire a double insu face au placebo." Presse Med., 15(31), 1556-8, 1986.
15. Clairambault, P., Magnier, B., Droy-Lefaix, M.T., Magnier, M., & Pairault, C., "Effet de l'extrait de ginkgo biloba sur les lesions induites par une photocoagulation au laser a l'argon sur la retine de lapin." Sem. Hop. Paris, 62, 57, 1986.
16. Le Poncin-Lafitte, M., Martin, P., Lespinasse, P., & Rapin, J.R., "Ischemie cerebrale apres ligature non simultanee des arteres carotides chez le rat: effet de l'extrait de ginkgo biloba." Sem. Hop. Paris, 58, 403, 1982.
17. Peter, H. "Vasoactivity of ginkgo biloba preparation." 4th Conf. Hung. Ther. Invert. Pharmacol., Soc. Pharmacol. Hung., B. Dumbovith, ed., 177, 1968.
18. Vilain, B., De Feudis, V. & Clostre, F. "Effect of an extract of ginkgo biloba on the isolated ileum of guinea-pig." Gen. Pharmac., 13, 401, 1982.
19. Auguet, M., De Feudis, V., Clostre, F. & Deghenghi, R. "Effects of an extract of ginkgo biloba on rabbit isolated aorta." Gen. Pharmac., 13, 225, 1982.
20. Auguet, M., De Feudis, V. & Clostre, F. "Effects of ginkgo biloba on arterial smooth muscle responses to vasoactive stimuli." Gen Pharmac., 13, 169, 1982.
21. Auguet, M. & Clostre, F. "Effects of an extract of ginkgo biloba and diverse substances on the phasic and tonic components of the contraction of an isolated rabbit aorta." Gen. Pharmac., 14, 277, 1983.
22. Etienne, A., Hecquet, F. Clostre, F. & De Feudis, F.V. "Comparison des effects d'un extrait de ginkgo biloba et de la chloropromazine sur la fragilite osmotique, in vitro, d'erythrocytes de rat." J. Pharmacol (Paris), 13, 291, 1982.
23. Racagni, G., Brunello, N. & Paoletti, R. "Neuromediator changes during cerebral aging. The effect of ginkgo biloba extract." Presse Med., 15(31), 1488-90, 1986.
24. Taylor, J.E. "Liasions des neuromediateurs a leurs recepteurs dans le cerveau de rats. Effet de l'administration chronique de l'extrait de ginkgo biloba." Presse Med., 15(31), 1491-3, 1986.
25. Auget, M., Delaflotte, S., Hellegourarch, A. & Clostre, F. "Bases pharmacologiques de l'impact vasculaire de l'extrait de ginkgo biloba." Presse Med., 15(31), 1524-8, 1986.
26. Mussgang, G. & Alemany, J. "Untersuchungen ueber periphere arterielle durchblutungstoerungen. XV. Mitt. Zur problematik der konservation behandlung obliterierender peripherer durchbluntungstoerungen, dargestellt an tinktur und extrakt aus ginkgo biloba L." Arzneimittel Forschung, 18, 543, 1968.
27. Trounier, H. "Klinish-pharmakologische untersuchungen ueber den effect eines

extraktes aus ginkgo biloba L. beim post thrombotischen syndrom." Arzneimittel Forschung, 18, 551, 1968.

28. Gautherie, M, Bourjat, P., Grosshans, E. & Quenneville, Y. "Effet vasodilateur de l'extrait de gingko biloba mesure part thermometrie et thermographie cutanees." Therapie, 27, 881, 1972.

29. Massoni, G., Piovella, C & Fratti, L. "Effets microcirculatoieres de la ginkgo biloba chez les personnes agees." Giorn. Geront., 20, 444, 1972.

30. Piovella, C. "effetti della ginkgo biloba sui micorovasi della congiuntiva bulbare." Minerva Med., 64, 4179, 1973.

31. Auguet, M. et. al., op. cit., 1986.

32. Galley (Yatley?), P. & Safi, N. "Tanakan et cerveau senile. Etude radiocirculographique." Bordeaux Med., 10, 171, 1977.

33. Bauer, U. "6-month double blind randomized clinical trial of ginkgo biloba extract versus placebo in two parallel groups in patients suffering from peripheral arterial insufficiency." Arzneimittel Forschung, 34, 716, 1984.

34. Hemmer, R. & Tzavellas, O. "Zur zerebralen wirksamkeit eines pflan-zenpraparates aus ginkgo biloba." Arzneimittel-Forschung, 17, 491, 1967.

35. Montanini, R. & Gaspari, G. "Impiego di un estratto di ginkgo biloba (TEBONIN) nella terapia delle vasculopatie cerebrali." Min. Card., 17, 1096, 1969.

36. Boudouresques, G., Vigourous, R., Boudouresques, J. "Interet et place de l'extrait de ginkgo biloba en pathologie vasculaire cerebrale." Medicine Praticienne, 55-75, 1975.

37. Moreau, Ph. "Un nouveau stimulant circulatoiere cerebral." Nouv. Presse. Med., 4, 2401, 1975.

38. Haan, J., Reekermann, V., Welter, F.L., Sabin, G. & Muller, E. "Ginkgo biloba flavonglykoside. Therapiemoglichkeit der zerebralen insuffizienz." Medizinische Welt, 33, 1001, 1982.

39. Eckmann, F. & Schlag, H. "Kontrollierte doppelblind--studie zum wirksamkeits-nachweis von tebonin forte bei patienten mit zerebrovaskularer insuffizienz." Fortschritte der Medizin, 100, 474, 1982.

40. Dalet, R. "Essai du tanankan dans les cephalees et les migraines." Vie Medicale, 35, 2971, 1975.

41. Daniel, F. "Les troubles trophiques d'origine veineuse des membres inferieurs, et leur traitement par le ginkor." Immex, Janvier, 1972, p. 129.

42. Locatelli, G.R. & Sorbini, E. "Effetto del tebonin (estratto delle foglie di ginkgo biloba l.) nel trattamento dell'arteriopatia periferica senile." Min. Card., 17, 1103, 1969.

43. Sorbini, E. "La ginkgo biloba nella terapia vascolare." Minerva Med., 64, 4201, 1973. 44. Natali, J. & Cristol, L. "Experimentation clinique d'un extrait de ginkgo biloba dans les insuffisances arterielles peripheriques." Vie Med., 16, 1023, 1976.

45. Ambrosi, C. & Bourde, C. "Nouveaute therapeutique medicale dans les arterio-pathies des membres inferieurs: tanakan. Essai clinique et etude par les cristaux liqui-des." Gaz. Med. France, 82, 628, 1975.

46. Garzya, G. & Picari, M. "Trattamento delle vasculopatie periferiche con una nuova sostanza estrattiva il tanakan." Clin. Europ., 20, 936, 1981.

47. De Amicis, E. "Attivita della ginkgo biloba nelle otopatie da arteriosclerosi." Minera Med., 64, 4193, 1973.

48. Lallemant, Y. & Barrier, M. "Etude d'un vasoregulateur d'origine vegetale en therapeutique O.R.L." Gaz. Med. France, 82, 3153, 1975.

49. Artieres, J. "Effets therapeutiques du tanakan sur les hypoacousies et les acou-phenes." Lyon Mediter. Medical, 14, 2503, 1978.

50. Natalie, R. Rachinel, J. & Pouyat, P.M. "Le tanakan dans les syndromes cochleo-vestibulaieres relevant d'une etiologie vasculaiere. Traitement de long cours." Gaz. Med. France., 86, 1381, 1979.

51. Haguenauer, J.P., Cantenot, F., Koskas, H. & Pierart, H. "Traitement des troubles

de l'equilibre par l'extrait de ginkgo biloba. Etude multicentrique a double insu face au placebo." Presse Med., 15(13), 1569-72, 1986.

52. Claussen, C.F. "Interet diagnostique et pratique de la craniocorpographie dans les syndromes vertigineux." Presse Med., 15(31), 1565-8, 1986.

53. Meyer, B. "Etude multicentrique randomisee a double insuface au placebo du traitement des acouphenes par l'extrait de ginkgo biloba." Presse Med., 15(31), 1562-4, 1986.

54. Dubreuil, C. "Essai therapeutique dans les surdites cochleaires aigues. Etude comparative de l'extrait de ginkgo biloba et de la nicergoline." Presse Med., 15(31), 1559-61, 1986.

55. Parnaud, E. "Ginkor en proctologie courant. A propos de 36 observations." Therapeutique, 47, 483, 1971.

56. Nora, J. "Place et interet de ginkor dans le traitement des affections hemorroidaires." Med. Chir. Dig., 3, 437, 1974.

57. Soullard, J. & Conton, J.F. "Experimentation du ginkor en proctologie." Sem. Hop. Paris, 54, 1177, 1978.

58. Gessner, B., Voelp, A. & Klasser, M. "Study of the long- term action of a ginkgo biloba extract on vigilance and mental performance as determined by means of quantitative pharmaco-EEG and psychometric measurements." Arzneimittel-Forschung, 35(9), 1459-1465, 1985.

59. Hindmarch, I. & Subhan, Z. Clin. Pharmacol. Res., 4, 89, 1980. 60. Hindmarch, I. "Activite de l'extrait de ginkgo biloba sur la memoire a court terme." Presse-Med., 15(31), 1592-4, 1986.

61. Pidoux, B. "Effets sure l'activite fonctionnelle cerebrale de l'extrait de ginkgo biloba. Bilan d'etudes cliniques et experimentales." Presse Med., 15(13), 1588-91, 1986.

62. Taillandier, J., Ammar, A., Rabourdin, J.P., Ribeyre, J.P., Pichon, J., Niddam, S. & Pierart, H. "Traitement des troubles du vieillissement cerebral par l'extrait de ginkgo biloba. Etude longitudinale multicentrique a double insu face au placebo." Presse Med., 15(31), 1583-7, 1986.

63. Clostre, F. "De l'organisme aux membranes cellulaires: les differents niveaux pharmacologiques de l'extrait de ginkgo biloba." Presse Med., 15(31), 1526-38, 1986.

64. Dehen, H., Dordain, G. & Allard, M. "Methodologie d'un essai controle dans la maladie d'Alzheimer." Presse Med., 15(31), 1577-82, 1986.

65. Allard, M. "Traitment des troubles du vieillissement par extrait de ginkgo biloba." Presse Med., 15(31), 1540-5, 1986.

66. Warburton, D.M. "Psycho-pharmacologie clinique de l'extrait de ginkgo biloba." Presse Med., 15(31), 1595-604, 1986.

67. Felber, J.P. "Effet de l'extrait de ginkgo biloba sure les parametres biologiques endocrines." Presse Med., 15(13), 1573- 4, 1986.

Ginseng
(panax ginseng)

The World's Best Anti-Stress Tonic

Guaranteed Potency Constituents.

Ginsenosides. The complex taxonomy and chemistry of ginseng make its standardization a difficult problem. Which kind of ginseng should be chosen? Which fractions of ginseng should be standardized? The answer to the first question involves deciding between the numerous plants that go by the name ginseng. One approach is to standardize extracts from them all. But there must be a starting point. The logical place to begin is with the most ancient and most clearly recognized species — panax ginseng. This should be differentiated from *panax quinquefolium* or American ginseng, *eleutherococcus senticosa* or Siberian ginseng, *panax japonicum* or Japanese ginseng, and from other plants less universally known as ginsengs: Brazilian, Alaskan, Patagonian, Himalayan, and so forth. Future standardizations should and will probably be made for the other species of ginseng.

The second question involves deciding which chemical fraction should be standardized. Official ginseng contains two main classes of saponins call ginsenosides: 1) derivatives of protopanaxadiol: $Rb1$, $Rb2$, Rc and Rd (hereafter called the $Rb1$ group); and 2) derivatives of protopanaxatriol: $Rg1$, Re, Rf, and $Rg2$ (hereafter called the $Rg1$ group). Most of the physiological properties of ginseng can be attributed to these groups. Since some of the actions of $Rb1$ are almost diametrically opposed to the actions of $Rg1$, we need to decide which fraction is most important; which fraction do we want to *guarantee* will be present at a certain level? To answer those questions we need to compare the properties of panax ginseng to those of the other major ginsengs. It is not as hard a task as it may appear.

Whereas American ginseng contains almost exactly the same sets of principles as the official ginseng, it does so in significantly different proportions. For example, both species contain the $Rg1$ group, but the panax species contains much greater amounts than the American ginseng. The $Rb1$ group predominates in both species, but is present in much greater quantities in the American species. Thus, the *Rb1/Rg1 ratios* are significantly different in the two plants. This distinction in levels of Rg1 accounts for observed differences in action between the American and the official ginseng. Siberian ginseng contains no ginsenosides at all; its action depends upon an entirely different set of saponins and polysaccharides. These differences are discussed in detail later on. For now, it is sufficient to observe that the most logical course of action in the standardization process, is to emphasize the *differences* between the species. Since both the American and the panax species contain Rb1, but only the panax contains appreciable Rg1, a good standardized panax ginseng will contain guaranteed amounts of the Rg1 fraction. Standardized American ginseng would conversely probably guarantee a certain level of Rb1 ginsenosides.

There are two ways to approach standardization. One is to produce a high potency extract. The other is to guarantee the levels of certain constituents as they would occur naturally in the whole herb. Based upon considerations such as cost-effectiveness and the possibility of unknown synergisms, I feel that the best *panax ginseng* product should be of the second kind, utilizing the best roots available. As long as the Rb1/Rg1 ratio is adequate, a less expensive, more effective product can be made from whole prime root, than from costly extracts of run-of-the-mill roots and rootlets. I recommend a standardized panax made from the roots of the Korean variety of *p. ginseng*, because the roots of this variety contain higher levels of the Rg1 fraction than any other species of ginseng. The root contains a characteristic profile of ginsenosides and contains all of the principle active constituents of the herb, including those not yet identified. Guaranteed Potency whole root of high quality will contain 4 percent ginsenosides in the form of Rg1 which will not be less than 50 percent of the Rb1 content (proprietary *extracts* advertising 10-14% ginsenosides are available, but in encapsulated quantities of a little more than 100 mg.; the product I discuss here should be available in 500 mg. capsules, at less cost!).

A guaranteed potency ginseng will, therefore, potentiate the Rg1 effects as much as possible and guarantee them at a certain constant level; this ensures reliable physiological activity. In the past, and even today, imported ginseng suffered and suffers horrendously from adulteration, improper attention to cultivation and harvesting procedures, the use of immature roots and rootlets and so forth. The Rg1 fraction is much more sensitive to production practices than the Rb1 fraction. Without knowing why, tradition has always demanded that extreme, almost fanatic, care be taken in all aspects of the production of the very best ginseng. Perhaps such measures have to do with protectingthe sensitive and highly prized Rg1 fraction. Perhaps in no other instance is the Guaranteed Potency concept better applied than in the case of ginseng.

History.

The reader is referred to any of the several currently available books that describe the history of ginseng in detail; In the interest of space, that history will not be needlessly reviewed again here.

Method of Action.

Overview

In the section on Guaranteed Potency Constituents, we differentiated between the Rb1 and Rg1 fractions, the two fractions commonly believed to contain most of the biological activity.

(A) The main pharmacological effects of the Rb1 group (highest in American ginseng) are as follows (alcohol soluble extract):

1. *central nervous system depressant : anticonvulsant, analgesic, tranquilizing*
2. *hypotensive*
3. *anti-stress — as demonstrated in the protection of the gut against stress-induced ulcers*
4. *antipsychotic: inhibition of conditioned avoidance response*
5. *weak anti-inflammatory response*
6. *antipyretic (fever-reducing)*
7. *facilitates small intestinal motility*
8. *increases synthesis of cholesterol in liver*
9. *increases RNA activity in rat's liver, though Rc has opposite effect;*

(B) The corresponding effects for the Rg1 group (highest in panax ginseng) are as follows (water soluble):

1. *slight central nervous system stimulant; activates brain activity as measured by EEG over occipital and sensorimotor areas; facilitates evoked potentials and conditioned reflexes*
2. *hypertensive*
3. *antifatigue*
4. *enhanced mental acuity, intellectual performance*
5. *anabolic: stimulates DNA, protein and lipid synthesis in bone marrow; may be responsible for observations of increased body weight and enhanced resynthesis of glycogen and high energy phosphate compounds; increases RNA and DNA content of adrenals and lymph nodes*

(C) There are other properties of panax ginseng that have not been clearly identified with either the Rg1 or Rb1 fractions. Some of these are also contradictory in nature.

1. *stimulates the immune system*
2. *impedes hypertrophy and atrophy of adrenals*
3. *reduces blood sugar level when it is high*
4. *raises blood sugar level when it is low*
5. *lowers white blood cell count when it is high*
6. *raises white blood cell count when it is low*
7. *has similar effects on red blood cell count*
8. *antidiuretic effect*
9. *heals deformities of the cornea, esp.* recent *cloudy opacities*
10. *exerts some anti-tumor effects*
11. *some positive effect on male sterility*
12. *some female (estrogenic) hormonal activity*

In surveying the relative concentrations of Rg1 and Rb1 fractions in different ginseng species, one observes that only panax ginseng contains enough Rg1 to impart the properties listed under (B) above. To these we might add an unknown portion of group (C). Without the Rg1 fraction, only group (A) (and some portion of group (C)) effects will be possible, and there exists the possibility that without Rg1 effects the plant loses its ability to be classified as a tonic (or adaptogen); its action will all be one way, so to speak. All known effects of panax ginseng will be present in the ginseng discussed in this chapter.

The contradictory properties of the various individual fractions of ginseng are what a tonic is all about. (There are those who might argue that a tonic pushes all in one direction — toward increasing the overall "tone" of the body, bringing it back from a state of lassitude, "stimulating" it. But my observations are that herbs generally listed as tonics push both ways. They only stimulate when stimulation is needed. Their action tends toward homeostasis.) The body takes what it needs from the plant, ignoring everything else. Theoretically, a body in perfect health would derive no benefit from a single exposure to ginseng or any other tonic.

For example, although it might seem that the sedative and stimulant properties of ginseng are contradictory, in fact the CNS depressant action, as expressed in ginsenoside Rb1, will be most active only when one is overly irritated or tending in that direction; and the CNS stimulant property will come into play only during severe stress. Each fraction's action is mediated by the action of the other fraction — so to speak. The proper Rg/Rb balance guarantees that the appropriate tonic response will be induced. The trick in producing a truly superior

Guaranteed Potency ginseng is getting the Rg concentration up where it belongs.

As was true in the History section, there are plenty of competent reviews of the mechanisms of action of ginseng; another one is not needed. In this chapter I will simply try to illustrate what difference the guaranteed level of Rg1 makes. I maintain that widespread discontent with *panax ginseng* products ensues from a dramatic variability in the concentration of the Rg1 fraction. With biologically meaningful amounts of that fraction guaranteed, important physiological processes, that depend on sensitive interactions among the ginseng constituents, are made possible.

Learning/CNS effects

Ginseng saponins are able to affect learning curves. In studies where rats were trained to climb a pole or jump over a barrier whenever a tone sounded, to avoid a mildly annoying foot shock, animals pretreated with Rg1 or with a lipid soluble fraction (roughly equivalent to Rb1) responded more rapidly to the tone stimulus than did controls.[1] In a follow-up study utilizing the same two techniques, neither substance significantly affected the initial learning of the tasks. But when the animals were forced to learn to discriminate between two similar sounds (one meaning 'jump' and the other meaning 'not-jump') the Rg1 treated rats were significantly better able to learn this discrimination.[2] In fact the Rb1-treated animals showed a slight depression in learning ability.

One of the most internationally respected ginseng research teams, from Japan, has done a lot of work with Rg1 and Rb1; they have provided much insight into stimulant and antifatigue properties of Rg1 and the sedative properties of Rb1.[3] They found that the mildly stimulating Rg1 fraction was effective in increasing the ability of rats to learn a simple Y-maze. A Y-maze is an alley-way that branches into right and left alleys on the other end. Learning is measured as the number of trials required before the rat learnes which alley contains food reward. The influence of Rg1 was determined by several variables that influenced how fast the animal will run to the reward. Rg1 significantly shortened the running time, while caffeine (a control substance) significantly lengthened the running time. Thus Rg1 facilitated the learning process, but in a manner different from and better than the more common stimulant, caffeine.[4] Similar effects were obtained by the same research team under other conditions.[5]

Several researchers have reported observing distinct but slight CNS stimulating activity, attributable to Rg1 in whole panax ginseng.

Reviews of that work are available.[6-8]

In humans, the Rg1 fraction of ginseng may be responsible for the increased capacity for mental work, as well as intellectual performance, observed in some studies.[9] Some studies report no noticeable increase in the volume of work, but rather a reduction in the number of errors or mistakes made. Other studies see both an increase in production and in accuracy.[10]

The anti-fatigue property of Rg1 has also been verified in experimental trials. For instance, in one study Rg1 accelerated the recovery from fatigued states in mice exposed to 4 hours of continuous work.[11] The authors reasoned that this could also indicate a CNS-stimulant activity. Some researchers believe, however, that the effects of ginseng on behavior, learning and fatigue so closely resemble the effects on those parameters of the common hormones ACTH and corticosteroids, that ginseng's effects may in fact be less the result of a direct action on the neurons than of the result of the herb's affect on the production and metabolic fate of the hormones.

The presence of choline in ginseng presents an interesting problem. It appears to be present in both water soluble (Rg1) and lipid soluble (Rb1) extracts. Choline performs many functions in the body. Besides being part of the synthetic pathway for lipids, it is crucial to proper neural functioning. Choline lowers the blood pressure, as would be expected from Rb1, but is an intrinsic part of the parasympathetic nervous system, the nervous system that mediates maintenance and normative factors in the body. Research has shown that dietary choline has important effects on mental capacity such as would be expected from Rg1. Choline, like Rb1, appears to have antipsychotic effects, but, like Rg1, appears to improve memory in patients suffering from senility. Therefore, the presence of choline will potentiate the general tendencies of either fraction.

Stress

When a person is exposed to any kind of stress, certain metabolic demands are made on the body. Central to the body's ability to respond appropriately, adapt to stressors, is the health and proper functioning of the adrenal gland. Adrenal-mediated cellular behavior will make the difference between survival and death, vitality and disease. It has been theorized that ginseng affects the body's response to stress in several ways. Mainly, ginseng increases the body's ability to restore homeostasis even as its metabolism is being upset by stress. What the reader needs to keep clearly in mind is that *both fractions are required in order for these processes to take place. The direction of action depends upon whether more emphasis is required from anabolic versus metabolic cellular events.* Both anabolic and metabolic processes will be affected, but you will experience conservation of energy and the building up of stores of proteins and lipids, adrenal hormones, etc., on one occasion, and the rapid and efficient use of energy stores on another. So important are these effects, that a special term has been created just to describe them: adaptogen.

In its broadest sense, according to the famous Soviet ginseng researchers, Lazarev, and Brekhman and Dardymov, an adaptogen is anything that "increases the nonspecific resistance of an organism" to stress and other detrimental environmental influences. Brekhman further limits the class of adaptogens to agents which (1) are nontoxic, and (2) normalize bodily processes,irrespective of the direction of the pathological changes, e.g., both hypo- and hyperglycemia should be normalized by an adaptogen. Further, "one of the most important indices of the action of adaptogens was their capacity to increase efficiency both after a single (stimulant action) or prolonged (tonic action) administration."[12]

In other words, an adaptogen is anything that behaves like ginseng. This may strike the reader as somewhat circular reasoning — that's because it is: an adaptogen is ginseng, and ginseng is therefore an adaptogen. One might ask why a substance has to be "nonspecific" when there are plenty of substances that increase adaptability in a very specific manner. Why must adaptogens be restricted to substances that can have observable effects after a "single" administration? So long as adaptation is increased, what difference does it make how many administations are required? And is there something wrong with a substance that only "normalizes" in one direction? Essentially, what the Russians did was list all of the properties of ginseng, eleutherococcus and related species, and used these descriptions as the definition of an adaptogen. The rigors of Western science demand that the properties of a new class of agents be delineated *independent* of data specific to a single substance. This procedure was clearly violated by Brekhman and colleagues. And, of course, the history of science demonstrates that labeling of this nature side-steps the necessity for analyzing the fundamental merits of the research itself.

What the labeling of ginseng as an adaptogen did do was to popularize ginseng in the public eye. It made discussion of the herb easier; it conveyed a definite feeling of authenticity and respectability, without the necessity of addressing technical material. The Russians proclaimed, "We have discovered a new wonderful class of agents, and ginseng is one." That, of course, sounds a lot better than, "We have discovered ginseng, and it is one." But the latter statement is truer.

A much better, more theoretically and scientifically sound approach would have been the incorporation of ginseng research into the model of stress then accepted by the medical world: The General Adaptation Syndrome of Hans Seyle, first announced in 1936. While the rest of the world's research on stress and anti-stress agents evolved and evolves within the general context of the G.A.S. and its derivatives, the little world of ginseng, and its fellow adaptogens, sat and sits in relative obscurity, spinning around dumbly, all by itself. That not only makes it difficult to evaluate positive research results, but makes it almost impossible to deal meaningfully with negative findings. For example, what do we do with studies that fail to observe "adaptogenic" effects.[13] There is not space here to rewrite the history of ginseng within a more fitting context — that will keep for a later publication. But the reader is advised to demand better explanations for ginseng's effects than, "it does this because it is an adaptogen."

With that in mind, let us see some of the ways ginseng affects metabolism and thereby mediates stress reactions.

ATP. Cellular respiration takes place within the cell in small bodies called *mitochondria*. They serve as miniature "power plants" that produce the energy needed for life. Through respiration, energy is transferred from carbohydrates and other food molecules to *adenosine triphosphate* (ATP), which is stored up and used by the cell to perform work. Rg1 would be expected to increase the cell's ability to produce and store ATP; Rb1 would be expected to increase the body's ability to utilize ATP when stress occurs.

Mitochondria are believed to produce a series of four chemical reactions to create ATP. The first involves an enzyme called ATPase, whose activity is directly facilitated by ginseng.

Liver. The liver plays a primary role in metabolism. Amino acids from foods are utilized by the liver to serve the body as a source of chemical energy. Much of this energy is used by the muscles where lactic acid accumulates; the blood transfers the lactic acid to the liver for resynthesis into glucose. This process depends largely on the activity of small intracellular structures composed of protein and RNA, called *polysomes*. Changes in the RNA of liver cells results in different rates of metabolism.

Ginseng has been shown to increase the rate of synthesis of RNA in the nucleus and cytoplasm of rat liver cells.[14] It also precipitates a rise of 46-49% in the synthesis of protein in the blood, especially albumin and gamma-globulin.[15] A single injection of certain saponins of ginseng increases the activity of a substance which helps produce RNA. Also, the increase of amino acid incorporation within the liver is 85% more active than in normal control animals.[16]

Changes in the liver induced by ginseng have been shown to enhance the synthesis of cholesterol. Particularly active in this synthesis was Rb1. The Rb1 also increased the rate cholesterol was excreted in bile and feces. Ginseng was shown in several studies to increase the incorporation of fats in the liver, coupled with slight decreases in blood sugar levels.[17] The authors suggested that ginseng increased the conversion rate of sugars into the necessary substrates for the formation of fatty lipids (accelerated lipogenesis). Several studies have shown that ginseng elevates plasma HDL levels, while lowering the LDL levels, a significant trend toward improved fatty acid balance.[18-19] Significant improvement in the plasma of human patients suffering from hyperlipemia has also been observed.[20]

Other researchers, utilizing a standard research procedure, found that rat liver, treated with ginseng extract, produced an increase in the incorporation of radioactive-labeled precursors into nuclear and cytoplasmic RNA and DNA-dependent RNA polymerase activity. Ginseng, administered directly into the stomach, caused an increase in the rate that serum proteins, such as albumin and gamma-globulin, are created.[21-23] The endoplasmic reticulum, the part of the cell most involved in metabolism, increased after four weeks. Other Japanese researchers discovered that the Rb1 fraction enhanced RNA polymerase activity in a manner similar to that produced by growth hormone and corticosterone.[24] Incidentally, the Rc component of the Rb1 fraction *repressed* polymerase activity; this indicates the presence of a tonic mechanism within the Rb1 fraction by itself.

This research seemed to offer a reasonable explanation for the increase in RNA and protein synthesis. Since a great majority of liver cell ribosomes and polysomes are usually bound in endoplasmic reticular membranes, an increase in endoplasmic reticulum would result in a marked increase in the metabolic capacity of the liver cells. The tonic action of panax ginseng might be explained, therefore, by enhanced RNA synthesis, changed polysome content, and enhanced endoplasmic reticulum and protein synthesis.

These results suggest that ginseng has a tonic effect because it increases the body's ability to utilize energy at the basic level. Changes in RNA content, ATPase activity and increases in endoplasmic reticulum in animals, after prolonged ingestion of ginseng, suggest that the plant simply increases the efficiency of the body's own natural metabolic processes. There are many plants that enhance the body's ability to function normally. That is what herbal medicine is all about. But ginseng, and other so-called adaptogens, as well as several plants that nobody yet includes in this elite circle, act upon some of the absolutely critical organs, glands and tissues of the body.

Adrenal/Pituitary Axis

Anxiety, anger, fear and physical danger, as well as exposure to severe temperature gradients and to prolonged overextension of physical capacity, will all cause stress reactions in the body. Prolonged stress probably helps to initiate such diseases as ulcers, high blood pressure, and asthma. Exposure to severe prolonged stressful situations can even result in tissue damage to the pituitary/adrenal stress mechanism of the body.

Hormones of the adrenal cortex (the outer part of the adrenal gland) are steroids controlled by a substance originating in the pituitary gland called adrenocorticotropic hormone (ACTH). The amount of ACTH and the amount of adrenal steroids increases in response to physical or emotional stress, to help the body cope or adjust. The steroids are the original "adaptogen," if you will; they change the response of the body to injury, and increase the amount of energy available to the cells. They have been shown to even increase the rate of learning.

The major organs involved in the stress system of the body are the hypothalamus (a nucleus of the brain), the pituitary (a gland attached to the base of the brain), and the adrenal glands deep within the body. Under stress, the hypothalamus signals the pituitary gland to produce ACTH. ACTH circulates in the blood, informing the adrenals to begin producing their hormones. These substances then help the body's cells adapt to the stress. They also signal the hypothalamus to stop telling the pituitary to produce ACTH, and, in the absence of ACTH, the adrenals cease to produce their hormones. The entire process is called a negative feedback system and operates very much like your home's thermostat.

Studies have shown that physiological changes due to stress are mediated, prevented, and reversed by the action of ginseng. When control animals are exposed to stress, changes are seen in the weight of several organs: adrenals, thymus, spleen and thyroid.[25-28] These changes are significantly inhibited by ginseng. Other physiological measures of stress are also inhibited. The physiological effects can be observed on a gross level in behavioral measures. For example, compared to controls, mice exposed to various experimental models of stress while being fed ginseng extract exhibit much less aggression, lower mortality, less fatigue, and so forth.[29-30]

One of the primary targets of ginseng activity is the adrenal itself. When the adrenals are removed, animals no longer respond to the administration of ginseng — it no longer has an effect on those physiolological actions that it affected while the adrenals were present, as measured by the animals' ability to tolerate temperature stress.

Of course, ginseng's effects are felt on more organs than just the adrenals, but adrenal effects are of special interest in the mediation of stress mechanisms. Over the years many hypotheses have been suggested to explain the action of ginseng saponins on the adrenal/pituitary axis. Gradually, one idea has gained ascendence over the others. This theory asserts that ginseng acts primarily and directly at the level of the pituitary and/or hypothalamus. Supporting research has shown that both Rb and Rg ginsenosides, when injected into the stomach cavity, produce an almost instant rise in plasma ACTH and adrenal corticosterone concentrations. A chemical known as dexamethasone blocks ACTH and so corticosterone secretion (by interrupting the feedback mechanism: if there is no circulating ACTH, then the adrenals cannot be induced to secrete hormones); the site of action of dexamethasone is known to be the pituitary and the hypothalamus. Now, what happens when you administer both ginseng and dexamethasone? If ACTH levels do not rise, then one can conclude that ginseng was unable to overcome the inhibitory effect of dexamethasone. And what does it mean if the ginseng-induced rise in circulating corticosterone is not seen? Since dexamethasone does not inhibit adrenal function, an absence of significant increases in corticosterone would mean that ginseng is not affecting the adrenals in a direct manner at all, that, in fact, ginseng must influence the adrenal *indirectly* by first stimulating the release of ACTH. The above scenario is exactly what was found in a series of experiments.[31-33]

Further evidence comes from the finding that ginseng increases plasma concentrations of adrenal-produced cyclic AMP (cAMP) in normal rats, but not in animals with the anterior pituitary gland removed.[34] This means, of course, that ginseng exerts its effects on cAMP levels *indirectly* via some intermediate action on the pituitary gland.

However, the action of ginseng is not as simple as the above arguments would make it sound. There is evidence that ginseng *does* have some direct effects on the adrenal glands. Ascorbic acid content in the adrenals varies inversely with the degree of stress: the more stress, the less ascorbic acid. In non-stressed animals, ginseng does not affect ascorbic acid levels, but when animals are subjected to heat or cold stress, ginseng initially accelerates the depletion of ascorbic acid, and then greatly helps to restore ascorbic acid in the adrenals.[35-36] Translating that into meaningful language, we can say that ginseng does seem to have a direct effect on the adrenals, because it helps the adrenals respond to stress by increasing the utilization of ascorbic acid stores, and then helps the adrenals recover from stress, and get ready for subsequent stress, by contributing significantly to stores of ascorbic acid in the gland. Ginseng has the same effect in animals with the pituitary gland removed, using ACTH as the stressor,[37] so it can not be acting indirectly on the adrenals via a primary affect on the pituitary gland. This finding provides strong evidence that ginseng is acting directly on the adrenals themselves. However, it does not exclude the possibility that ginseng may simply be affecting the normal metabolic fate of circulating adrenocortical hormones (and ACTH) so as to perpetuate their activity.[38] Other research has shown that ginseng inhibits experimentally-induced adrenal atrophy (and thymus atrophy);[39] this finding also implies a direct effect on the adrenals.

The adrenal-related research weakens hypotheses that attribute the anti-stress action of ginseng solely to its ability to stimulate the release of ACTH via some direct influence on the central nervous system.[40-41] The emphasis is thereby shifted from the Rg1 fraction to the Rg1/Rb1 ratio.

Stephen Fulder has presented an attractive synthesis of much of the experimental data on ginseng.[42] He favors the hypothalamus/pituitary axis as the primary site of action of ginseng, noting that the bulk of the evidence supports the notion that ginseng interferes with the normal feedback control of adrenal corticoid levels. He suggests that the mechanism of action involves a *sensitization* of hypothalamic cell membranes to the effects of stress; this would encourage the passage of adrenal corticoids into the cell and bring about the typically quick and potent response of the adrenals caused by ginseng.

Stress-related studies, carried out mainly by the Russians and the Chinese, have shown that ginseng facilitates healing, has definite anti-inflammatory effects, prevents an increase in white blood cells in the circulatory system, is antipyretic, weakens the symptoms of chronic gastritis and elevates the appetite, stimulates immune-system function, and heals ulcers.

Korean scientists have proven that ginseng increases the number of protective cells in the gastrointestinal lining of mice, even after stress. Ginseng accelerated the DNA synthesis in stomach (epithelial) cells in normal mice and promoted recovery in stressed animals. Similar results have been obtained for cells in the trachea, lymph glands, adrenal gland, liver and pancreas. We will return to considerations of stress adaptation in the next section.

Cardiovascular and digestive effects

Two of the traditional uses of ginseng, both in the Orient and in North America, have been for the stomach and for the heart. Research has supported the use of ginseng to improve digestion, inhibit cholesterol absorption, but increase cholesterol synthesis, and lower the level of cholesterol circulating in the blood. It is felt that the latter finding results from ginseng-induced increases in the metabolic and catabolic conversion of cholesterol into steroid molecules. Ginseng also decreases the amount of nonsaturated and saturated fatty acids in blood serum.[43-44] But evidence for an even more direct action is available. For example, it is known that ginseng directly suppresses arrhythmias.[45] Other cardiovascular effects, such as lowered heart rate, lowered blood pressure and arterial pressure, have been reported.[46-47]

Modern Chinese doctors still recommend ginseng for heart failure in its early stages. For shock and hypotension, ginseng is said to improve heart functioning and to elevate blood pressure. Research has, in general, supported these uses. Ginseng has also been found to improve the blood supply to the brain, probably through dilating the vessels of the pia mater (the membranes surrounding the brain). The herb increases iron uptake in the blood and the amount of oxygen used, andretards the production of experimentally-induced renal hypertension.

Other effects

This review cannot begin to cover the myriad, experimentally substantiated, effects of ginseng. Several properties are not reviewed here simply because they are only partially affected by the Rg1/Rb1 ratio: antidiuretic, cornea-healing, anti-tumor, anti-shock, estrogen, anti-toxic (radiation, poisoning, etc.), anti-inflammatory, cell-mediated immunity, fertility, geriatrics, and respiratory distress, to name a few. These properties are no less important, and may be even more important, than those reviewed, but space considerations simply do not allow a comprehensive treatment in this book.

Therapeutic Research and Action.

As was true in the History and Method of Action sections, I will not present an exhaustive review of all the studies bearing on clinical and practical effects of ginseng. The reader is probably already familiar with these properties, and if not, may find extensive reviews elsewhere (including a forthcoming book by the author and colleague on the subject). Instead, I will make some general comments to help the reader evaluate research on ginseng, and then I will present a simple summary of effects one can expect from the use of ginseng.

Problems in evaluating ginseng research

As the reader may have noticed in the previous pages, the Japanese have provided much careful and systematic research on a preclinical level, while the Russians have provided the bulk of the research on a therapeutic or clinical level. Japanese research is detailed and logically concise, and the researchers seldom speculate beyond their data. Russian research is, at times, questionable: Not only is it sometimes methodologically imprecise, thereby allowing other valid interpretations of results, but, on occasion, the authors use the pages of journals to propagandize. Such misuse of science cannot help but cast doubt on research results which conveniently support party lines, and would lead unerringly to the world- wide distribution of soviet products. The reader would do well to find corroborating research before making definitive evaluations of Soviet-directed research.

Research on humans is, of course, difficult to control, analyze and draw conclusions from. There are obvious ethical questions involved in using human subjects, plus there is the ever-present and difficult to control placebo effect. The latter problem is especially difficult in regards to ginseng, since most people bring to its use a plethora of expectations. For example, in a case reported in the British Medical Journal, a woman patient taking ginseng reported increased sexual desire. There are, however, two equally logical and equally likely explanations. First, ginseng may increase sexual desire. Second, the patient thought that ginseng should increase sexual desire. With sexual desire, you would expect the same result either way.

Russian researchers were the first to experimentally confirm the tonic effects of ginseng, though the plant had been used for this purpose for centuries. The perception of well-being and increased vigor are created by the metabolic effects of the plant. Dosage level may be important. At least one study has reported that small dosages are stimulant, but large dosages may be sedative.[48]

Therapeutic actions of panax ginseng

A. Following is a list of physiological effects to be expected by the routine consumption of standardized ginseng with an Rg1/Rb1 ratio of at least 50%.

1. *Increased mental acuity, which should be revealed in better memory, better intellectual performance, increased reaction time, greater volume of work (on certain tasks), and better subjective feelings.*
2. *Increased tone throughout the cardiovascular system, including the heart , arteries and veins.*

3. *Increased production of DNA; may be responsible for increased learning potential.*

4. *Increased endurance; anti-fatigue action.*

5. *Increased life-span; anti-radical and antioxidant effects.*

6. *Anabolic effects which lead to accelerated production of DNA, as well as protein and lipid synthesis.*

7. *Anti-cancer effects.*

8. *Some stimulating effect on the immune-system similar to, but perhaps more gentle than, that expected from Rb1.*

9. *Some mild aphrodisiac action. Ginseng has been shown to increase fertility, but the aphrodisiac action, although it may involve increased glandular health, is still best explained as a placebo effect.*

B. Following is a list of physiological effects that would also be expected from the guaranteed potency ginseng discussed in this chapter, but which rely heavily on the Rb1 component. These effects will probably not be experienced except when the homeostasis of the body is sufficiently upset to require their normalizing action. The following effects would also likely be seen at any time in a standardized American ginseng extract.

1. *Sedative and tranquilizing actions, including depressed reaction time and slower rates of learning.*

2. *Hypotensive effect on cardiovascular system, i.e., lowered blood pressure.*

3. *Anti-toxin action; radioprotective action; ability to protect against nitrogen and mustard gas poisoning.*

4. *Increased RNA production, which increases metabolism and the production of proteins such as antibodies.*

5. *Anti-convulsant activity; able to partially counteract the effects of strychnine.*

6. *Stimulation of body's immune system by increasing the production of antibodies in the bone marrow.*

7. *Anti-inflammatory, antipyretic and analgesic actions.*

8. *Enhanced synthesis of cholesterol and the breakdown of cholesterol into other steroids; eventually leading to a slight reduction in blood sugar levels.*

9. *Enhanced resistance to temperature-induced stress and noise-induced stress.*

Based in part on the physiological properties listed above and in part on the mass of clinical data gathered over the past 30 years or 3,000 years, depending on how reliable you consider ancient Chinese medicine, one may expect good therapeutic effects from ginseng in the treatment of the following conditions.

This is the ginseng "Top Twenty."

1. Cancer	11. Stress
2. Diabetes	12. Asthma
3. Radiation Sickness	13. Headaches
4. Neurosis	14. Anemia
5. Hypotension	15. Indigestion
6. Hypertension	16. Impotence
7. Arthritis	17. Depression
8. Cardiac arrythmia	18. Nervousness/Anxiety
9. Atherosclerosis	19. Menstrual Disorders
10. Fatigue/Exhaustion	20. Heart Disease

Following is a list of additional indicated uses for ginseng.
1. To increase learning and memory capacity.
2. To increase work performance.
3. To increase life span & counteract the natural aging process.
4. To enhance the body's natural immunity.
5. To increase sexual appetite and vitality.
6. To accelerate convalescence.

Route of Administration.

Ginseng products have been administered several ways: whole root, tinctures, tablets, teas, capsules, cigarettes, injections, chewing gum, candy and snuff. Several of these preparations reflect questionable efforts to somehow get a "buzz" from the herb, and are strongly discouraged.

This Guaranteed Potency preparation is available only as an encapsulated powder. Teas can be made from it without any change in efficacy (just be sure to ingest the residual powder).

Dosage.

An appropriate dosage is difficult to ascertain. Generally, it will depend on individual tastes and needs. That may seem like a pretty vague recommendation, but it is hard to be more specific. The following suggested doses are, therefore, to be considered as highly arbitrary.

Daily Tonic: 1-3 capsules/day
For Acute Stress: 3-6 capsules/day
For Chronic Stress: 2-5 capsules/day

I have heard it suggested, and I tend to agree, though without any real scientific justification, that year-round use should be avoided. The idea is to provide the body with regular periods of time wherein it can adjust its own physiology to changing biochemical, biological and environmental conditions. As I discuss in the next section, a healthy stress-free body may view ginseng as a stressor, rather than as an anti-stress agent.

Toxicity.

First of all, panax ginseng is a tonic. Any reports of toxicity are therefore suspect, by definition. That is, either a few thousand years of usage to establish the tonic character of panax ginseng are wrong, or something is wrong with the reports of toxicity.

Following is a list of common deficiencies in reports of toxic reactions to ginseng: 1) It wasn't panax ginseng. In today's market where the lure of big money is automatically attached to ginseng, there is a definite risk of fraud. Substances that have definitely been shown to not be panax ginseng (or any form of ginseng) have been sold as such. Other adulterations are possible. 2) Other substances were included with the panax ginseng, and the toxic reaction was due to these. Panax is quite often adulterated by totally worthless plant materials and/or addicting stimulants. 3) Prior conditions were identified only after ginseng use began. There are probably other problems, but these three account for most "false positive."

One report of toxicity, for example, appeared in the British Medical Journal. A 70-year old woman developed swollen, tender breasts, with diffuse nodularity, purportedly as the result of taking ginseng for three weeks. She also experienced a general sense of "well-being." Breast symptoms disappeared after cessation of ginseng. Two successive trials with ginseng produced the same result.[49] The indictment here appears strong, but must be evaluated in the context of the woman's total physical condition, particularly in relationship to the condition of her hormonal system. At 70 years of age, there is a more than good chance that she was suffering from prior conditions of which she might not have been totally aware, malfunctions in the endocrine system that modified her response to ginseng. The tonic action of the herb may have been temporarily obscured by these factors. Since we are told nothing about the rest of the woman's physical condition, it is impossible to evaluate this possibility. Also the question "What would have happened as a result of continued use?" remains unanswered. We are also not told if the woman was taking other drugs simultaneously with ginseng. Could ginseng chemicals have been modified by other drugs or diet? Could the action of other drugs have been modified by ginseng? Was it truly panax?

And, of course, we must say something about Ronald Siegel's invention: The Ginseng Abuse Syndrome. Again, space will not allow an extended discussion of Siegel's work, but some comments must be made in way of perspective. First of all, although Siegel fails to substantiate his claims, there really may be ways to abuse ginseng. Persons, under no stress whatsoever, may experience some adrenal stress from prolonged used — that hasn't been demonstrated, but it is an hypothesis that arises naturally from the body of research on ginseng and the theoretical work of Hans Seyle. It especially applies to American ginseng. But, Siegel does not differentiate between panax and other species.

Second, just because Siegel's article appeared in the pages of the Journal of the American Medical Association, that does not indicate anything about the validity of his presentation. JAMA will print almost anything anti-herbal without review, without hesitation.

Third, the procedural errors of Siegel's methods completely invalidate his project and provide no glimmer of reliability for his conclusions. Although he collected a lot of information, he made no effort to control any confounding variables whatsoever. Reading his report reminds one of the state of pre-Newtonian science in which there were volumes upon volumes of raw data exhibiting no unifying direction or theoretical focus, awaiting the arrival of somebody to make sense of it, separate the meaningful from the obtuse. When Newton finally did that, it required some application of the scientific method. The Ginseng Abuse Syndrome, unlike the Opticks, apparently does not need scientific validation. One might ask Siegel, for example, upon what basis he can assert that hypertension, nervousness, sleeplessness, skin eruptions and morning diarrhea can be attributed to ginseng, when the people were simultaneously using caffeine? Out of 133 people recruited (how and where and from what population?), 14 were diagnosed as exhibiting Ginseng Abuse Syndrome (was this syndrome identified before, during or after the study?). Is that a statistically significant number? Where are the individual case histories (two are partially given)? He states that those who *injected* ginseng were eliminated from the study, but in one of the two partial case histories the person is reported to have injected 2 ml of an extract in order to produce psychotropic effects.

But perhaps the most glaring shortcoming of the study, the one which removes it from the realm of science, is the failure to include a control group of subjects matched to the experimental group in as many ways as possible (age, sex, job-type, health, etc.), with the exception that no member of the control group be allowed to use ginseng. This simple (and required) procedure may have helped determine (by subtraction) what residual effects could be attributed to ginseng and to nothing else. Without this necessary provision, the results of the study can reasonably be attributed to intervention of any one of many confounding variables. Research that ignores the most basic experimental procedures is usually done in the interest of a "cause," for personal gain.

More traditional tests of toxicity have shown that the herb is extremely safe to use in any absolute sense. In fact, it is probably best described as an anti-toxic substance. The lengthy discussion provided here is required in view of the many sources for misinformation that exist concerning ginseng. Another factor is the common distribution of fraudulent products. And yet another determinant is simply the large number of people using ginseng. All of these combine to cloud the issue. In the final analysis, reliable research trials have established many subtle mechanisms of action for panax ginseng, and very little toxicity at either therapeutic doses or at much larger doses. The standardized Guaranteed Potency product, recommended in this chapter, will hopefully provide an avenue for avoiding most of the traditional problems encountered in preparing, buying and using panax ginseng.

References.

1. Saito, H., Tsuchiya, M., Naka, S. & Takagi, K. "Effects of panax ginseng root on conditioned avoidance in rats." Japanese Journal of Pharmacology, 27, 509-516, 1977.
2. Saito, H., Tsuchiya, M., Naka, S. & Takagi, K. "Effects of panax ginseng root on acquisition of sound discrimination behaviour in rats." Japanese Journal of Pharmacology, 29, 319- 324, 1979.
3. Takagi, K. "Pharmacological studies of some oriental medicinals." Yakhak Hoeji, 17(1), 1-8, 1973.
4. Takagi, K., Saito, H. & Tsuchiya, M. Japanese Journal of Pharmacology, 24, 41-48, 1974.
5. Takagi, K, Saito, H. & Nabatoa, H. "Pharmacological studies of panax ginseng root." Japanese Journal of Pharmacology, 22, 245-259, 1972.
6. Petkov, V.W., "Ueber den wirkungsmechanismus des panax ginseng C.A. Meyer." Arzneimittel-forschung, 11, 288-295, 1961.
7. Brekhman, I.I. & Dardymov, I.V. "Pharmacological study of ginseng and related plants." Proc. Pacific Sci. Congr., 11th, 8, 11, 1966.
8. Kim, E.C., Cho,H.Y. & Kim, J.M. "Effect of panax ginseng on the central nervous system." Korean J. Pharmacol., 2, 23-28, 1971.
9. Popov, I.M. & Goldwag, W.J. American Journal of Chinese Medicine, 1, 263-270, 1973.
10. Fulder, S. About Ginseng, Thorsens Publishers, New York, 1984, p. 29.
11. Saito, H., Yoshida, Y. and Takagi, K. "Effects of panax ginseng root on exhaustive exercise in mice." Japanese Journal of Pharmacology, 24, 119-127, 1974.

12. Brekhman, I.I. & Dardymov, I.V. "New substances of plant origin which increase non specific resistance." Annual Review of Pharmacology, 9, 419-430, 1969.
13. See, for example, Lewis, W.H., Zenger, V.E. & Lynch, R.G. "No adaptogen response of mice to ginseng and eleutherococcus infusions." Journal of Ethnopharmacology, 8(2), 209-214, 1983.
14. Hiai, S., Oura, H., Tsukada, K. & Hirai, Y. Chem. Pharm. Bull., 19, 1656, 1971.
15. Oura, H., Hiai, S., Odaka, Y. & Yokozawa, J. Biochem. (Tokyo), 77, 1057, 1975.
16. Oura, H., Hiai, S., Nabetani, A. Nakagawa, H., Kurata, Y. & Sasaki, M. Planta Medica, 28, 76, 1975.
17. Yokozawa, T., Seno, H. & Oura, H. "Effect of ginseng extract on lipid and sugar metabolism. I. Metabolic correlation between liver and adipose tissue." Chem. Pharm. Bull. (Tokyo), 23, 3095-3400, 1975.
18. Yamamoto, M., Uemura, T, Nakama, S., Uemiya, M. & Kumagi, A. "Serum HDL-cholesterol-increasing and fatty liver-improving actions of panax ginseng in high cholesterol diet-fed rats with clinical effect on hyperlipidemia in man." American Journal of Chinese Medicine, 11(1-4), 96-101, 1983.
19. Qureshi, A.A., Abuirmeileh, N., Din, Z.Z., Ahmad, Y. & Burger, W.C. "Suppression of cholesterogenesis and reduction of LDL cholesterol by dietary ginseng and its fractions in chicken liver." Atherosclerosis, 48(1), 81-94, 1983.
20. Yamamoto, M. et. al., op. cit., 1983.
21. Oura, H., Hiai, S., Nakashima, S. & Tsukada, K. Chem. Pharm. Bull., 19, 453, 1971.
22. Oura, H., Hiai, S., Odaka, Y. & Yokozawa, T. Journal of Biochemistry, 77, 1057, 1975. 23. Hiai, S., Oura, H., Tsukada, K. & Hirai, Y. Chem. Pharm. Bull., 19, 1656, 1971.
24. Iijima, M & Higashi, T. "Effect of ginseng saponins on nuclear ribonucleic acid (RNA) metabolism. II. RNA polymerase activities in rats treated with ginsenoside." Chem. Pharm. Bull., 27(9), 2130-2136, 1979.
25. Brekhman, I.I. "Pharmacological investigations of glycosides from ginseng and eleutherococcus." Lloydia, 32(March), 46-51, 1969.
26. Brekhamn & Dardymov, op. cit., 1969.
27. Petkov, V. & Staneva-Stoicheva, D. "The effect of an extract of ginseng (panax ginseng) on the function of the adrenal cortex." In Chen & Mukerji, Eds., Pharmacology of Oriental Plants., Oxford, Pergamon Press, 1965, pp. 39-50.
28. Kim, J.Y. "Influence of panax ginseng on the body weights of rats." Korean Journal of Physiology, 4, 1-4, 1970.
29. Banerjee, U. & Izquierdo, J.A, "Antistress and antifatigue properties of panax ginseng: comparison with piracetam." Acta Physiol. Lat. Am., 32(4), 277-285, 1982.
30. Wang, B.X., Cui, J.C., Liu, A.J. & Wu, S.K. "Studies on the anti-fatigue effect of the saponins of stems and leaves of panax ginseng." Journal of Traditional Chinese Medicine, 3(2), 89-94, 1983.
31. Hiai, S., Yokoyama, H., Oura, H. & Yano, S. "Stimulation of pituitary-adrenocortical system of ginseng saponin." Endocrinol. Japon., 26(6), 661-665, 1979.
32. Petkov & Staneva, op. cit., 1963.
33. Bohus, D. & Strashimirov, D. Neuroendocrinology, 6, 197, 1970.
34. Hiai, S., Sasaki, S. & Oura, H. "Effect of ginseng saponin on rat adrenal cyclic AMP." Planta Medica, 37, 15-19, 1979.
35. Petkov & Staneva-Stoicheva, op. cit., 1965.
36. Kim, C., Kim, C.C., Kim, M.S., et. al. "Influence of ginseng on the stress mechanism." Lloydia, 33, 43-48, 1970.
37. Kim, C., et. al., op. cit., 1970.
38. Zhang, S.C. & Jiang, X.L. "The anti-stress effect of saponins extracted from panax ginseng fruit and the hypophyseal- adrenal system." Yao Hsueh Hsueh Pao, 16(11), 860-863, 1981.

39. Tanizawa, H., Numano, H. Odani, T., Takino, Y., Hayashi, T. & Arichi, S. "Study of the saponin of panax ginseng C.A. Meyer. I. Inhibitory effect on adrenal atrophy, thymus atrophy and the decrease of serum K+ concentration induced by cortisone in unilateral adrenalectomized rats." Yakugaku Zasshi, 101(2), 169- 173, 1981.

40. Petkov, V. & Staneua, S. "The effect of an extract of ginseng on the adrenal cortex." Proceeding of the 2nd International Pharm. Meeting in Prague, 1963, Pergamon Press, Czech Med. Press, Vol 7: 39-45.

41. Petkov, W. & Staneva, D. "Der einfluss eines ginseng-extraktes auf die funktionen der nebennierenrinde." Arzneimittel-Forschung, 13, 1078, 1963.

42. Fulder, S.J. "Ginseng and the hypothalamic-pituitary control of stress." American Journal of Chinese Medicine. 9(2), 112-118, 1981.

43. Sakakibara, K, Shibata, Y, Higashi, T., Snada, S. & Shoji, J. Chem. Pharm. Bull.(Tokyo), 23, 1009, 1975.

44. Namba, T., et. al. "Hemolytic and its protective activity of ginseng saponins." Chem. Pharm. Bull., 21, 459-461, 1973.

45. Zhang, R.B., Li, Z.Y. & Shi, H.T. "Cardiac arrhythmia induced by hypothalamic stimulation in cardiac ischemic rabbits and the antiarrhythmic action of panax ginseng." Chung Kuo Yao Li Hsueh Pao, 3(4), 226-230, 1982.

46. Chen, X. "Experimental study on the cardiovascular effects of ginsenosides." Chung Hua Hsin Hsueh Kuan Ping Tsa Chih, 10(2), 147-150, 1982.

47. Lee, D.C., Lee. M.O., Kim, C.Y. & Clifford, D.H. "Effect of ether, ethanol and aqueous extracts of ginseng on cardiovascular function in dogs." Canadian Journal of Comprehensive Medicine, 45(2), 182-187, 1981.

48. Hong, S.A., Park, C.W., Kim, J.H., Chang, H.K., Hong, S.K. & Kim, M.S. Korean Journal of Pharmacognosy. 10, 1-11, 1974.

49. Palmer, B.V., Montgomery, A.C.V., Monteiro, J.C.M.P. "Gin Seng and mastalgia." British Medical Journal, 13 May 1978, p. 1284.

Milk Thistle

(silybum marianum l. gaertn. or carduus marianus l.)

For The Liver

Guaranteed Potency Constituents.

Silymarin and related flavonoids. Since 1954 we have known that milk thistle contained flavonoids. But it wasn't until the mid '60's that researchers discovered the unique chemistry of these flavonoids. A group of three of the most potent flavonoids — silybin, silydianin & silychristin — are known collectively as *silymarin*. Silymarin, at the time of its discovery, constituted a whole new class of compound, and its amazing properties continue to astound the scientific world. Since silymarin is practically insoluble in water, it remained for science to produce a compound that would lend itself easily to both medical research and human consumption. Today, the better standardized milk thistle extracts are manufactured only by sophisticated European labs. The best are guaranteed to contain 80% silymarin in a natural base.

The differences between using the extract and simply ingesting whole seed are those of potency and guarantee. Whole seed cannot be guaranteed to contain a given amount of flavonoids. One cannot be sure what a handful of seed actually represents. This is not a problem unless you have a liver disease — then you will want the higher potency of the extract, and you will want it guaranteed.

History.

Milk thistle is numbered with the most ancient known herbal medicines. Theophrastus and Dioscorides recommended the root mixed with honey as a cough medicine. Pliny, in about 100 A.D. named the plant silybum (meaning thistle); however, he treasured the plant for its nutritional, rather than its medicinal, value. During the Middle Ages, probably through the migration of monks, milk thistle was brought to middle and northern Europe. There, the folk history of this weed becomes really interesting. Growing as it did, mostly in the gardens of churches and cloisters, it was prized by monks and nuns and took on several different metaphysical, mystical and religious connotations. Another common name for milk thistle is Maria thistle, a name that reflects its Middle Age heritage. Other ancient names for the plant include Christ's Crown, Heal Thistle, Venus Thistle, "The Wand of God's Grace," and so forth. The herb was feared as much as it was prized by the common people. It is said that this thistle could not be stored over an oven or it would cause the members of the household to argue and fight constantly. Milk thistle can be observed in many of the paintings of that era, especially in those of the Virgin Mary and the martyrs.

Lonicerus, in 1564, was the first physician to report using silybum (crushed seeds) to treat liver disorders; namely, inflammation. In 1626 Matthiolus listed similar indications and recommend milk thistle especially as a diuretic and for getting rid of kidney stones. Somewhat later, in 1755, Von Haller mentioned his practice of using milk thistle for all liver disorders. From that time forward (except for an extended period during the 18th century), milk thistle became a standard agent of choice in the liver therapeutics of European physicians. Other medical doctors of the Middle ages included milk thistle in their written materia medica. Among them were Hieronymus Bock (1595), Jacobus Theodorus (1664), Adamo Lonicero (1679) and Valentini (1719).

The hiatus of the 18th century ended when Johannes Gottfried Rademacher rediscovered the usefulness of milk thistle. In 1848, near the end of his brilliant career, Rademacher was able to provide a fairly detailed list of liver ailments and the particular milk thistle preparations best suited for treatment. He discussed chronic liver disease, acute hepatitis, spleen disorders, and jaundice. His research solidified the medicinal use of milk thistle in the medical literature.

Moving to this century we find Schulz, in 1919, recommending milk thistle for female complaints of uncertain origin and vague symptomology located generally in the vicinity of the upper part of the colon and the liver, and also for cases of gall stones. Virtually every important European pharmacopoeia of this century recommended milk thistle for disorders of the liver, gall bladder and spleen.

Developments in folk medicine directly paralleled the progress that was being made in the medical area. The seed of the milk thistle was commonly used as a cholagogue, to promote the flow of bile, as a tonic for the spleen, gallbladder and liver, for jaundice from any cause. The fruit, or seed, was also used for indigestion, dyspepsia, lack of appetite and other stomach and/or digestive disorders. In homeopathy, the folklore uses were repeated: a tincture from the seeds was used for liver disorders presented as jaundice and/or gallstones; the seeds and leaf were also used for peritonitis, coughs, bronchitis, uterine congestion and varicose veins. A fine bitter tonic was sometimes made from the leaf, but most laymen realized that the greatest portion of medicinal activity was concentrated in the seed. It has been said that milk thistle was at one time used as a substitute for ergot alkaloids in the treatment of metrorrhagia and menorrhagia. Most of these folk uses persisted into modern times and are currently popular in the folk medicine of most European and North American countries.

Method of Action.

While clinical physicians of the early 1900's were treating a wide variety of liver disease, research physicians carried out numerous laboratory experiments, designed to elucidate the various mechanisms of action. One of the earliest published reports (1931) established the ability of milk thistle to stimulate the flow of bile.[1] This action helped to explain why milk thistle was so effective in the treatment of indigestion and other disorders of the digestive system. However, compared to some of the other herbs discussed in this book, milk thistle is not one of the best digestive aids or cholagogues. In fact, its cholagogue property is not strong enough to account for its many beneficial effects on the digestive system. More basic kinds of studies need to be carried out in this area before we will obtain a satisfactory understanding of milk thistle's action.

Subsequent to the discovery that milk thistle (Mte) provided significant protection to the liver against several kinds of potent toxins, research on the substance exploded. Hundreds of studies were carried out, a small sampling of which are presented here. Because that body of research, especially the pre-clinical stuff, tends to utilize a group of standard experimental routines and procedures, I have based the following discussion on some of the most common research models used.

Common research methods

Carbon tetrachloride

The administration of a combination of carbon tetrachloride and hexobarbital is one of the most common methods for assessing the ability of a substance to protect the liver against the effects of harmful chemicals. The reasoning is as follows. Hexobarbital produces reliable and consistent patterns of sleep in experimental animals. The normal length of sleep per dosage level has been carefully worked out in normal animals. Any observed deviation in sleep time reflects some disturbance in underlying physiology, which, in this case, is the ability of the liver to metabolize the narcotic. Any increase in sleeping time can be attributed to some impairment in the ability of the liver to break down the narcotic. Carbon tetrachloride produces such an impairment. The amount of impairment (read increase in sleeping time) per dosage level has also been carefully standardized in experimental animals. This procedure is important because it is used as a measure of liver functioning in human diagnostic medicine, especially in the differential diagnosis between obstructive and systemic jaundice.[2]

Against the backdrop of the dynamics outlined above, another substance, such as Mte is added. Will it increase or decrease sleeping time? Will it antagonize the effects of carbon tetrachloride, potentiate those effects, or have no influence at all? In the case of Mte, the increase in sleeping time normally produced by the carbon tetrachloride is dramatically reduced (60%).[3] This means that Mte effectively protects liver function from the toxic action of the poison.[4]

Another common procedure for determining the ability of a substance to protect liver function involves measurements of the liver's ability to metabolize p-oxyphenylpyruvic acid (OPH). OPH, produced during the degradation of tyrosine, is metabolized exclusively in the liver. That quantity of OPH which isn't metabolized in the liver is excreted in the urine. Therefore, the level of OPH in the urine increases following the administration of a liver toxin. Substances that counteract the toxin tend to bring urine OPH back to normal. Histological studies (the microscopic examination of thin slices of tissue) of the liver reveal how much structural damage the liver has incurred from administration of the toxin; histology therefore serves to substantiate chemical analysis. Since the histological picture resulting from carbon tetrachloride poisoning is very similar to that of hepatitis, this is another good reason for using this chemical in experimental studies. Following carbon tet administration, OPH levels in the urine increase dramatically. Mte again significantly counteracts the effects of the carbon tet, so much so, that the results are almost indistinguishable from controls.[5]

Some additional comments about the use of carbon tetrachloride may be of interest to some readers. Because of the simplicity and the reproducibility of effects inherent in the use of carbon tet, this procedure assumes particular importance. And, because this toxin is so often used, a continuous picture of its effects on the liver has been put together. By gradually increasing the dose, a reliable series of effects can be achieved, from fatty degeneration at the lower end, progressing through cellular death, fibrosis and cirrhosis. The functional correlates to the morphological signs are also well documented: from metabolic disturbances to a whole host of enzymatic changes both in the liver and blood.[6-7] For example, an increase in plasma enzyme concentration usually means that damaged liver cells are unable to contain the enzymes in a normal fashion; an increase in mitochondrial activity usually correlates with increased enzymatic activity, and so forth. The purpose of all this science is to create a body of information from which reliable generalizations to the human condition can be made. Such purposes must also be attributed to the use of all other experimental methods. The most popular of these methods relative to Mte are discussed below.

Amanita mushroom poisoning

One particular kind of experimental procedure has been very popular with researchers studying the properties of Mte. This procedure measures the ability of Mte to protect the liver against the effects of amanita poisoning. Amanita (death cap) is a very poisonous mushroom containing several different kinds of toxins, commonly divided into two groups:[8-9] the phallotoxins or phalloides, and the amanitoxins, which are collectively known as amanitine (though you can get more specific; e.g., there is alpha-amanitine; or you can get even more specific, e.g., alpha-amanitine is 2-hydroxyethyl-trimethyl-ammoniumhydroxide; we'll stick with amanitine). The manner in which the mushroom toxins kill was elucidated almost completely by 1960.[10]

The original amanitine studies were undertaken with the pre-conceived notion that Mte would have very little antagonistic effect, since few other toxins are as potent as amanitine (it causes severe hemorrhagic liver dystrophy and death within 2-5 hours); in addition, the researchers had to use very small animals as experimental subjects, since they didn't have enough Mte to meet the demands of larger heavier animals. Hence mice were used, and these creatures are particularly susceptible to amanitine toxicity. However, right from the first, it became obvious that Mte was an extraordinary hepatoprotective agent. Test results revealed a highly significant tendency for Mte to prevent, or at least inhibit, the effects of amanitine.[11] The early results were so impressive that chemical houses began to produce Mte in increasingly large amounts. This stimulus in production had two very beneficial consequences. First, it made possible research with larger creatures, including man; secondly, it provided the impetus for greater manufacturing output of products suitable for sale and use by people.

Over the past 20 years or so, researchers have exhibited a great deal of interest in the protective property of Mte against amanitine poisoning. Many different measures have been used and/or devised in the attempt to tease apart the mechanism of action.[12-13] One popular measure has been life span. Mte greatly increases lifespan in poisoned animals. Another measure is total body weight. Mte significantly inhibits the loss of weight normally observed in poisoned animals. Animals fed sub-lethal doses of amanitine normally lose weight very rapidly and gain it back very slowly. Animals fed a combination of amanitine and Mte lose weight much more slowly and gain it back much more rapidly.[14]

Another common measure of the ability of Mte to prevent amanitine damage is plasma sorbital-dehydrogenase (SDH) levels. SDH is a common liver-specific enzyme; plasma concentration of this enzyme is very small in healthy subjects (animals and humans). When damage to liver cells occurs, the concentration of SDH in plasma increases. Substances with hepatoprotective action will inhibit the rise in plasma SDH produced by certain toxins, in this case, amanitine. In the typical experiment, Mte is given on day one, and a combination of Mte and amanitine is administered on subsequent days. At some future point, the plasma SDH level of experimental animals is compared to that of controls (animals that received amanitine but no Mte). In these experiments, a great deal of variation in individual response is seen; the overall tendency is toward significantly lower SDH concentration in the experimental subjects, a finding that demonstrates the protective action of Mte.[15]

It should be noted that much of the research reviewed in this section has been replicated with the phallotoxins, and similar results have been obtained.[16-20]

Those readers with an appreciation for the ironies of applied research will be interested in the fact that carbon tetrachloride, that same toxin discussed in the previous section, markedly protects the liver against the effects of both amanitine and phallotoxin. Apparently it prevents the conversion of phalloidin to a toxic metabolite, and also prevents the binding of phalloidin to hepatocytes.[21]

Thioacetamide

Yet another experimental toxin commonly utilized in the study of the hepatoprotective role of Mte is thioacetamide (TAA). When TAA is fed to animals over a period of weeks to months, it produces liver damage that closely resembles that of cirrhosis in man. Eventually, death results from chronic administration of TAA. Three measures of

113

Mte effectiveness can be obtained from experiments using TAA. First, it should reduce the amount of liver damage, and second, it should increase the lifespan of experimental subjects. Both of these objectives are fully achieved. The third measure, that of body weight, is also affected; though Mte does not prevent weight loss due to TAA, it inhibits loss in a dose dependent manner.[22-24]

Other toxins

Mte effectively counteracts the toxic effects of several other kinds of poisons. For example, when the salts of rare earth metals (e.g., praseodymium, indium and cerium) are injected into lab animals, they characteristically induce hepatotoxic symptoms, such as necrosis (cell death) and steatosis (fatty degeneration). When subjects are pretreated with Mte, the toxic effects of the rare earths are greatly reduced, or prevented altogether.[25] In addition, Mte helps, in a therapeutic manner, to restore health to damaged cells. Although such research increases our understanding of the manner in which Mte works, it is not at all clear what it means for medicine and health. It would be interesting to know, for example, whether the frequent ingestion of Mte would protect the liver against the myriad daily encounters with heavy metals, free radicals and other environmental and dietary toxins. Research with praseodymium indicates that pretreatment with Mte may alter the kinetics of the metals thereby producing a more rapid elimination from the body. Alternatively, it may stimulate the formation of metal-binding proteins which, in turn, effectively detoxify the metals. Finally, Mte may inhibit the ability of the metals to bind with cells at receptor sites. Any of these mechanisms could come into play in the presence of toxins from whatever source. In one interesting study along these lines, Mte counteracted the effects of cadmium. Cadmium is an environmental pollutant that accumulates in human tissues over time, produces, among other things, hypertension, liver, kidney and neural damage, and hemorrhagic necrosis of the liver and testes. Pretreatment with Mte almost completely prevents mortality and hemorrhagic necrosis in the testes and liver, and reduces neuronal damage.[26]

A finding that hits closer to home involves the ability of Mte to partially counteract damage to the liver derived from the ingestion of alcohol.[27] Its effect, in this case, is not nearly as strong as it is against other toxins. However, on the clinical level, Mte is most effective in cases of cirrhosis that are caused by alcohol consumption.

In other, related, studies the hepatotoxic effects of the cold-blooded virus FV3 (Frog Virus 3) on warm-blooded animals is completely antagonized by Mte. The rationale behind such a strange choice of toxin is that it avoids some of the complexities of interpretation inherent in most viral-induced liver damage. Hepatitis induced by normal experimental viruses acts by multiplication of the virus particles in the liver. Therefore, substances counteracting such viruses must act by controlling multiplication; it is difficult to say what effect is being produced on liver cells themselves. Frog Virus 3, however, produces a purely toxic hepatitis; lesions are produced without multiplication of cells. In this model, the site of Mte action is directly on the cell structures themselves.[28]

Experimentally, amanita mushroom toxins, rare earths, carbon tet, and so forth, have been used as models, but there is no reason why the effects of Mte could not protect liver cells against other more common toxic substances. Certainly, the experimental findings support the traditional folklore uses of milk thistle seed in the treatment, prevention and cure of liver diseases of a wide variety. Every once in awhile one reads of the application of Mte in a clinical setting, in the treatment of miscellaneous poisonings. For example, two cases of severe food poisoning from toxins of flagellates were once reported. Both cases responded very rapidly to Mte, showing subjective, biochemical and histological improvements.[29]

Cellular mechanisms

Through the use of experimental methods, including those discussed above, scientists have discovered much about possible mechanisms of action of Mte. In mice and rats, Mte can reduce the lethality of amanita phalloides and amanitine from LD100 to LD0. Mte administered to mice within the first 30 minutes after poisoning, completely antagonizes the effects of the toxin — applied any later, and it doesn't; in one study using mice, if the treatment was withheld for 2 hours after amanita poisoning, no significant curative effects were observed.[30] In dogs Mte exhibits antidotal effects for up to 24 hours after poisoning.[31] Signs of intoxication appear in 8-10 hours and death occurs after 30-40 hours. It has been found that the mortality rate in mice injected with phalloides can be as high as 95%, but can be cut almost in half when treated with Mte.[32]

However, the toxic mechanisms and time course of the two amanita poisons are completely different. The Amanitoxins are thirty times more toxic than the phallotoxins but take substantially longer to work. Phalloides produce substantial toxicity within 2 hours (causing death within 5-8 hours), during which time they increase the permeability of liver cell membranes, thereby destroying them and releasing actin-containing components which, in turn, create openings in the membrane through which cytoplasm may protrude. Amanitine does not produce death in most cases until 3-7 days have elapsed. It acts by blocking protein synthesis. It penetrates the cell membrane to the nucleus where it inhibits polymerase B, without which messenger RNA cannot leave the nucleus. It follows that there can be no coding of ribosomal RNA, with the consequence that the cell can no longer produce protein. Once the current supply of protein is used up, the cell "starves" and then dies. Thus amanita toxins cause both morphological and enzyme-chemical toxic changes in cells.[33-37] Since Mte inhibits both types of toxins, it is likely that it exerts a primary effect on the cell membrane, ultimately stabilizing and strengthening that structure. In support of this concept is the finding that Mte and both poisons actively compete for the same cell membrane receptor sites.[38-45]

Also, in support of the above hypothesis, is research that systematically explores the effects of carbon tet and d-galactosamine on plasma level of several enzymes. The results again support the protective and curative properties of Mte, and have prompted authors to formulate several ideas about the possible roles Mte might play. They have postulated a mechanism by which Mte activates the regeneration of liver cells; in addition, they have suggested that Mte may act as an acceptor of radicals — a free-radical scavenger.[46-47]

There is some indication that the mechanism of action of whole death cap mushroom is qualitatively different from that of both subclasses of constituents alone. Most research focuses either on amanitine or on the phalloides. Because the mechanisms of action of the two toxins are so different, it simplifies things if the effects of each is studied separately. For this reason, there are very few studies that use an extract of the whole mushroom. However, the death rate and nature of the toxicity appears to be different when the whole mushroom is involved. One study reported 205 cases of clinical poisoning with whole death cap mushrooms. Death occurred in about 23% of all cases and in 51% of children under 10. The average period of time between ingestion and first clinical symptoms was 10 hours in those patients that died, and 2.6 hours for those that survived.[48] In one study, Mte was more effective than any other agent in preventing the toxic effects of a whole extract of amanita mushroom.[49] The fact that Mte is effective against both classes makes it an excellent choice for treatment, and suggests that perhaps more data along these lines are needed.

Interestingly, the mouse and rat cannot absorb amanita toxins orally; the toxins must be injected in order to produce toxicity. Dogs and humans not only absorb the poisons, they also develop a continuaous *enterohepatic* circuit. That means the toxins are cycled continuously between the gastro-intestinal tract and the liver (with some biliary excretion) increasing the amount of liver damage on each pass.[50] When Mte is administered to people in a clinical setting (meaning they have inadvertently or intentionally ingested amanita mushrooms), some length of time, usually quite long, has already gone by, yet there is still time to prevent death. This is because toxicity produced through an enterohepatic circuit usually takes considerable time to develop. The larger and heavier the organism, the longer it takes to produce toxicity. Once administered, Mte concentrates in the liver and quasi-interrupts the enterohepatic circuit. First it interrupts the primary absorption of toxins, and secondly it helps prevent their reabsorption due to enterohepatic circulation.[51] Cells not yet poisoned, are protected from damage from circulating alpha-amanitins, and act as centers for the generation of new liver cells.[52-57] With time, complete restoration of the liver is possible.

About 50% of orally administered Mte in humans is enterally absorbed and excreted unchanged or as a conjugate of glucuronic acid. Ten to twenty percent finds its way into the enterohepatic circuit. Since the Mte concentration is higher in the bile than in the blood, it is assumed that some kind of active or "uphill" transport mechanism is operative, and that Mte accumulates selectively in the liver. This would help explain the magnitude of the substance's effects on liver disease.[58-60]

One of the ways Mte accelerates the regeneration of destroyed liver tissue is by stimulating cellular protein synthesis. In studies wherein the livers of rats were partially removed, the administration of Mte promoted regeneration of liver tissue. The mechanism of action was the stimulation of nuclear polymerase A activity, which, in turn, stimulated ribosomal RNA and the subsequent generation of protein from which new cells could be built and nourished.[61-64]

Other cellular processes have been implicated in the therapeutic activity of Mte. For example, Mte inhibits lipoxygenase, one of the enzymes necessary for the damaging action that leukotrienes have on the liver. The inhibition of lipoxygenase disrupts the catalytic pathway by which oxygen and polyunsaturated fatty acids combine to form leukotrienes.[65-66] The possibility that Mte is a good free radical inhibitor also exists. Mte is essentially a flavonoid, and almost all flavonoids are good antioxidants or free-radical scavengers. As we learn more about the antiperoxidative functions of flavonoids, we may learn that these comprise the most important liver-protective mechanisms. Meanwhile, there is very little reason to doubt the research literature that overwhelmingly indicates that Mte inhibits free radicals.

Summarizing, the effectiveness of Mte is due to a combination of two primary mechanisms: First, it induces an alteration of cell membranes in such a way that only small amounts of toxins may penetrate into the cell; second, it accelerates the rate of protein synthesis, and thereby promotes cellular regeneration. While these are the two main processes, other, secondary, mechanisms such as free radical and lipoxygenase inhibition are probably involved.

It should be noted that the toxic effect of amanitine on the tubular epithelium of the kidneys is also blocked by Mte.[67] And there is research to indicate that the cellular tissues of the brain and other organs are also protected.[68-69]

Therapeutic Research.

Extensive clinical trials have clearly substantiated the ability of Mte to reverse the symptoms of many liver disorders, both acute and chronic, ranging from acute viral hepatitis to cirrhosis.[70-76] It stimulates liver cells to generate tissue to replace that which has been damaged or destroyed by disease. Although the liver already possesses such ability to a greater extent than perhaps any other organ of the body except the skin, that regenerative capacity slows down or ceases altogether when infected or damaged by alcohol or other drugs. Hence, the need for a medicine like Mte.

Amanita poisoning

More than half of all mushroom poisoning in man can be traced to the ingestion of amanita mushrooms. Most cases are lethal. Some clinical research has demonstrated that if the intoxication is diagnosed early enough, there exists a substantial chance for the victim's recovery following treatment with Mte. Lethality is reduced almost immediately after Mte treatment, and the rapidity of complete liver cell regeneration depends upon how far gone the liver was prior to treatment. The earlier Mte is administered, the more swiftly recovery takes place.

Liver disease

Mte has been very effective over a wide range of clinical manifestations of liver disease. While some of these trials have been almost anecdotal in nature, most have been well-controlled, double blind studies involving over 3,000 patients. Toxic-metabolic liver disease, acute viral hepatitis, chronic-persistent hepatitis, chronic-aggressive hepatitis, cirrhosis of the liver, fatty degeneration of the liver, and various liver disease of unknown etiology, are among the conditions investigated. The strongest positive effects have been observed in various forms of toxic-metabolic hepatitis (including alcohol-induced and iatrogenic, drug-induced forms), and in cirrhosis. Although Mte has no antiviral properties, it has been shown to shorten the course of viral hepatitis and to minimize post hepatitis complications.[77-90] Mte is even effective in protecting the liver against morphological and functional dysfunctions normally resulting from certain kinds of liver surgery.[91] Indications of improvement in the state of the liver are usually gathered, first in the form of subjective measures such as general condition, appetite, epigastric discomfort, enlargement and increased consistency of the liver, and second, from objective measurements usually based on blood plasma tests. For example, changes in membrane permeability are deduced from measurements of glutamic-pyruvic transaminase (GPT), glutamic-oxaloacetic transaminase (GOT), lactic acid dehydrogenase (LDH), sorbital dehydrogenase, and gamma glutamyl transpeptidase (GGT); membranotropic properties and the excretory functions of the liver are assessed through measurements of bilirubin, LAP, gamma-GT, alkaline phosphatase, and bromethalein; synthesizing ability is measured and assessed through prothrombin, triglycerides, and cholesterin; and measurements of mesenchymic activity include clotting factors, alpha, beta and gamma globulin, immunoglobulins IgA, and IgG.

Many, many studies could be reviewed, but most are simply replications and extensions of a simple and basic research approach: find patients with liver disease, administer Mte, watch what happens. Therefore, in the interest of space, just a couple of typical studies will be reviewed here. These should give the reader a general idea of how research on Mte goes forward. One (typical) study involved the participation of 129 patients for a period of about one month. The patients suffered from a number of different conditions, including obvious toxic or toxic-metabolic liver damage, fatty degeneration of the liver for various reasons, and chronic hepatitis. A control group of 56 patients was used for comparison. Mte significantly modified subjective and objective symptoms, stimulated a return to normal enzymatic activities, and improved digestive disorders (from the very first week). Enlarged livers diminished substantially in volume. A 50% regression in pathological symptoms, versus 25% in controls, occurred. And, no cases of intolerance, side effects, or allergic reactions were observed.[92] In another study, in an intensive follow-up situation, the long term beneficial effects of Mte therapy were observed in certain patients that were using Mte. Thirty-six patients with liver cirrhosis, chronic hepatitis and chronic aggressive and acute hepatitis were closely followed for several months. Good response was seen in acute hepatitis (including those forms involving cholestasis and serum hepatitis). The inflammatory process diminished or disappeared in cases of chronic aggressive hepatitis and liver cirrhosis.[93]

Therapeutic Action.

Liver disease

From the wealth of research on Mte reviewed in this chapter, it should be obvious that Mte is an excellent substance to use in the prevention and treatment of practically any liver disorder.

Poisoning, cirrhosis, hepatitis, fatty degeneration, necrosis, and so forth are all amenable to the use of Mte. The earlier the conditions are caught, the better the chances for complete recovery but effective treatment is possible at virtually every stage. Not only will Mte arrest the course of the disease, but it will stimulate individual liver cells to become sites for local regeneration of liver tissue. Over time, complete restoration of the liver is possible. Left alone the liver will, of course, self-regenerate. The point we wish to drive home is that the liver is seldom left alone. Its detoxification battle goes on continuously, 24 hours a day. Should the liver itself get sick, it's normally a long fight back to normal. At such times it is especially helpful to use Mte, for it can stimulate regeneration at four times the normal rate.

Daily living

The therapeutic importance of Mte extends beyond the very specific properties that formed the basis for much of the research carried out so far, such as its antidotal use in the presence of amanita poisoning. More importantly, the implications of the research heavily favor the idea that regular ingestion of Mte will provide a substantial amount of protection to the sick or healthy liver during the course of normal living. By stabilizing cell membranes, by encouraging the regeneration of cells destroyed during the normal detoxification process, Mte provides the liver and the body with the ability to triumph over the deleterious effects of daily encounters with air-, water-, and food-borne toxins.

Though Mte's role in the prevention of free radical and leukotrienes damage has not been fully elucidated, it is certain that the herb is active in this way. Combining Mte with other flavonoids would therefore comprise a terrific approach to liver protection.

Alcohol abuse

One of the uses for Mte that emerges from the literature is in stimulating the regeneration of tissue and function in the livers of persons subject to alcohol abuse. For instance, in one study we haven't yet reviewed, patients with fatty degeneration of the liver were divided into groups according to the cause of the condition (diabetes, obesity, alcoholism). Mte produced substantially better improvement in the group in which alcohol was either the sole, or one of the multiple causative factors.[94] We will undoubtedly see Mte used in alcohol treatment centers in this country in the not too distant future. Milk thistle should be in the daily diet of anyone recovering from alcohol abuse.

Drug abuse

The term 'drug abuse' may be too strong for what I have in mind, but it fits well within the concepts of wholistic medicine: namely, the use of prescription medicines, legally or illegally. Many psychopharmacologic drugs and agents are detoxified by the liver. During that process, liver cells die by the hundreds of thousands. The cumulative effect of drug use (abuse) on the liver can be devastating. Therefore, a wise course of action for those who want or need to take drugs is to supplement that intake with Mte. Milk thistle has been shown, experimentally, to prevent liver damage caused by psychopharmacologic drugs.[95]

Route of Administration.

Milk thistle extract is best administered orally in capsule form. There is no indication in the literature that i.v., i.m. or any other route is required or necessary for good therapeutic effects.

Dosage.

A wide range of dosages have been reported in the literature. Using a standardized 80% silymarin extract, a normal dose would be 3-6 175 mg capsules per day, taken with water before meals. Such a dose would substantially contribute to digestion and would, over a period of weeks and months, tend to restore normal metabolic activity and stimulate the regenerative activity of the liver.

In acute cases or in case of poisoning, dosages several times that recommended here have been administered without side effects, toxicity or allergic reactions.

Toxicity.

Original toxicity trials in mice, rats, guinea pigs and dogs, using different routes of administration, in acute, subchronic and chronic regimens, found that even very large doses of Mte were non-toxic and produced no side effects or allergic reactions.[96] Tests in humans also show that high doses of Mte are well-tolerated, both subjectively and as recorded by objective measurements.[97]

References.

1. Westphal, K. Gallenwegsfunktionen und Gallenleiden. Springer Verlag, Berlin, 1931, p. 326.
2. Koehler, P. Zhurnal Ges. Inn. Med., 19, 599, 1964.
3. Hahn, G., Lehman, H.D., Kurten, M., Uebel, H. & Vogel, G. "Zur pharmäkologie und toxikologie von silymarin, des antihepatotoxishcen wirkprinzipes aus silybum marianum (L.) Gaertn." Arzneimittel-Forschung, 18(6), 698-704, 1968.
4. Hahn, G., et. al., op. cit., 1968.
5. Hahn, G., et. al., op. cit., 1968.
6. Balazs, T. & Grice, H.C., Toxicol. Appl. Pharmacol., 5, 387, 1963.
7. Megirian, R. J. Pharmacol. Exp. Ther., 144, 331, 1964.
8. Floersheim, G.L. "Antagonistic effects against single lethal doses of amanita phalloides." Naunyn-Schmiedeberg's Archives of Pharmacology, 293, 171-174, 1976.
9. Wieland, Th. "Poisonous principles of mushrooms of the genus amanita." Science, 159, 946-952, 1968.
10. Matschinsky, F., Meyere, U. & Wieland, O. Biochem. Z., 333, 48, 1960.
11. Hahn, G. et. al., op. cit., 1968.
12. Vogel, G. & Trost, W. "Neutralization of the lethal effects of phalloidin and alpha-amanitin in animal experiments by substances from the seeds of silybum marianum L. Gaertn." Naunyn-Schmiedeberg's Arch. Pharmacol., 282, 109, 1974.
13. Floersheim, G.L. "Treatment of experimental poisoning by extracts of amanita phalloides." Toxicology and Applied Pharmacology, ü34, 499-508, 1975.
14. Hahn, G. et. al., op. cit., 1968.
15. Hahn, G., et. al., op. cit., 1968.
16. Obauer, G. & Schoen, H. Arzneimittel-Forschung, 14, 1257, 1960.
17. Vogel & Trost, op. cit., 1974
18. Vogel, G. & Trost, W. "Zur anti-phalloiden-activitat der silymarine silybin und disilybin." Arzneimittel-Forschung, 25, 392-393, 1975.
19. Frimmer, M. & Kroker, R. "Phalloidin-antagonisten. 1. Mitteilung. Wirkung von silybin-derivaten an der isoliert perfundierten rattenleber." Arzneimittel-Forschung, 25, 394-396, 1975.
20. Petzinger, E., Homann, J. & Frimmer, M. "Phalloiden-antagonisten. 2. Mitteilung. Protektive wirkung von disilybin beider vergiftung isolierter hepatozten mit phalloidin." Arzneimittel-Forschung, 25, 571-576, 1975.
21. Kroker, R. & Frimmer, M. "Decrease of binding sites for phalloidin on the surface of

liver cells during carbon tetrachloride intoxication." Naunyn-Schiedeberg's Arch. Pharmacol., 282, 109-111, 1974. 22. Hahn, G., et. al., op. cit., 1968.

23. Schriewer, H. Badde, R., Roth, G. & Rauen, H.M. "Die antihepatotoxische wirkung des silymarins bei der leberschaedigung durch thioacetamid." Arzneimittel-Forschung, 23, 160, 1973.

24. Schriewer, H.M. & Lohman, J. "Regulationsstoerungen des phospholipidstoffwechsel der gesamtleber, mitochondrien undmikrosomen bei der akuten intoxikation durch thioacetamid und deren beeinflussung durch silymarin." Arzneimittel-ÅForschung, 26, 65, 1976.

25. Strubelt, O., Siegers, C.P. & Younes, M. "The influence of silybin on the hepatotoxic and hypoglycemic effects of praseodymium and other lanthanides." Arzneimittel-ÅForschung, 30, 1690-1694, 1980. 26. Braatz, R. "The effect of silymarin on acute cadmium toxicity." In: Braatz & Schneider, op. cit., pp. 31-36, 1976.

27. Antweiler, H. "Effects of silymarin on intoxication with ethionine and ethanol. In Braatz & Schneider, op. cit., pp. 80-82, 1976.

28. Elharrar, M., Bingen, A., Drillien, R., Bendrault, J.L., Steffan, A.M., & Kirn, A. "Ein neues modell der experimentellen toxischen hepatitis. Die akute degenerative hepatitis der maus, ausgeloest durch das Frog Virus 3 (FV3)." Arzneimittel-Forschung, 30, 452-454, 1980.

29. Schopen, R.D. & Lange, O.K. "Beitrag zure therapie der haptosen--weiter beobachtungen zur therapeutischen anwendbarkeit von silymarin." Med. Welt, 15, 691, 1970.

30. Floersheim, G.L. op. cit., 1976.

31. Vogel, E., Trost, W., Mengs, U. & Sieck, R. Abstr. Proc. 7th Int. Congr. Pharmcol. Paris, 1978, p. 572, Pergamon Press, Ltd., Oxford.

32. Vogel, G. "Silymarin das antihepatotoxische wirkprinzip aus silybum marianum L. Gaertn., als antagonist der phalloidin-wirkung." Arzneimittel-Forschung, 1063, 1968.

33. Vogel, G., Trost, W., Braatz, R., Odenthal, K.P., Bruesewitz, G., Antweiler, H . & Seeger, R. "Untersuchungen zur pharmakodynamik, angriffspunkt und wirkungsmechanismus von silymarin, dem antihepatotoxischen prinzip aus silybum mar. L. Gaertn. I Mitt.: akute toxikologie bzw. vertraeglichkeit, allgemeine und spezielle (leber-) pharmakologie." Arzneimittel-Forschung., 25, 82, 1975. 34. Manganaro, M. & Di Cesare, L.F. "Fattori concorrenti alla rigenerazione del fagato dopo epatectomia parziale del ratto." Epatologia, 23, 245, 1977.

35. Wieland, O., "Changes in liver metabolism induced by the poison of amanita phalloides." Clin. Chem. (N.Y.), 2, 323-338, 1965. ì

36. Wieland, O., Fischer, H.E. & Reiter, M. ÇNaunyn-Schmiedeberg's Arch. Exp. Path. Pharmak., 215, 75, 1952.

37. Tyutyulkova, N., Gorantcheva, U., Tuneva, S., Chelinova-Lorer, H. "Effect of silymarin on the microsomal glyco protein and protein biosynthesis in liver of rats, with experimental galactosamine hepatitis." Methods Find. Clin. Pharmacol., 5, 181, 1983.

38. Weil, G. & Frimmer, M. "Die wirkung von silymarin auf die mit phalloidin vergiftete isolierte perfundierte rattenleber." Arzneimittel-Forschung, 20, 862-863,1970.

39. Vogel, G. & Temme, I. "Die curative antagonisierung des durch phalloidin hervorgerufenen leberschadens mit silymarin als modell einer antihepatotoxischen therapie." Arzneimittel-Forschung, 19, 613-615, 1969.

40. Vogel, G., Braatz, R. & Mengs, U. "On the nephrotoxicity of alpha-amanitin and the antagonistic effects of silymarin in rats." Agents Actions, 9, 221-226, 1979

41. Vogel, G. "The anti-amanita effect of silymarin." In: Faustlich, H., Kommerell, B. & Wieland, T. (Eds): Amanita Toxins and Poisoning, pp. 180-187. Witzstrock, Baden-Baden, New York, 1980.

42. Vogel, G. "Natural substances with effects on the liver." In: Wagner, & Wolff, P.

(Eds.): ÇNew Natural Products and Plant Drugs with Pharmacological, Biological or Therapeutical Activity, pp. 249-265, Springer Verlag, Berlin, New York, 1977.

43. Vogel, G. "Silymarin, das antiheptotoxische wirkprinzip aus silybum marianum L. Gaertn., als antagonist der phalloidin-wirkung." Arzneimittel-Forschung, 18, 1063-1064

44. Faustlich, Jahn & Wieland, üop. citü., 1980.

45. Frimmer, M. "Comparative studies on effects of silymarin in phalloidine action in perfused livers, isolated hepatocytes and isolated membrane systems." In: Braatz, R. & Schneider, C.C. (Eds): Symposium on the Pharmacodynamics of Silymarin, Cologne, Nov. 1974, pp. 13-19. Urban & Schwarzenberg, Berlin, 1976.

46. Rauen, H.M. & Schriewer, H. "Die antihepatotoxische wirkung von silymarin bei experimenÄtellen leberschaiedigungen der ratte durch tetrachlorkohlenstoff, d-galaktosamin and alakohol." Arzneimittel-Forschung, 21, 1194, 1971.

47. Rauen, H.M., Schriewer, H. "Enzymaktivitaetskorrelationen im serum nach experimenÄtellen leberschaedigungen der ratte." Arzneimittel-Forschung, 21, 1206, 1971.

48. Floersheim, G.L., Weber, O., Tschumi, P. & Ulbrich, M. "Die klinische knollenblaetterpilzvergiftung (amanita phalloides): prognotische faktoren und therapeutische massnahmen. (Eine analyse anhand von 205 faellen.) Schweiz. Medizinische WochenÅschrift, 112. 1164-1177, 1982.

49. Floersheim, G.L., op. cit., 1976.

50. Fauser, U. & Faustlich, H. "Beobachtungen zur therapie der Knollenblaetterpilzvergiftung. Verbesserung der prognose durch unterbrechung des enterohepatischen kreislaufs (choledochusdrainage)." Deutsche Medizinishce Wochenscrift, 98, 2259. 1973.

51. Faulstich, H., Jahn, W. & Th. Wieland, "Silybin inhibition of amatoxin uptake in the perfused rat liver." Arzneimittel-Forschung, 30(3), 452-454, 1980.

52. Flammer, R. "Hinweise auf silymarin bzw. silybin. Therapieempfehlungen bei knollenblaetterpilzvergiftungen." In Flammer, R. Differentialdiagnose der Pilzvergiftungen, pp. 17, 23, 24. G. Fischer, Stuttgart, New York, 1980.

53. Homann, J., Wizemann, V., Matthes, K.J. & Lasch, H.G. "Therapie der akuten "Knollenblaetterpilzvergiftungen." Hepatology, 12, 1522-1523, 1982.

54. Hruby, K., Lenz, K., Moser, C.D., Bachner, J. & Korninger, C. "KnollenÅblaetterpilzvergiftungen in Oesterreich." Wein. Med. Wschr., 91, 509-513, 1970.

55. Floersheim, G.L. "Treatment of experimental poisoning by extracts of amanita phalloides." Toxicol. Appl. Pharmacology, 34, 499-508, 1975.

56. Floersheim, G.L. "Antagonistic effects against single lethal doses of amanita phalloides." Naunyn-Schmiedebergs Arch. Pharmacol., 293, 171-174,1976.

57. Floersheim, G.L., Eberhard, M. Tschumi, P. & Duckert, F., op. cit., 1978.

58. Behrendt, W., Lorenz, D. & Mennicke, W.H. "Elimination of silybin in the bile collected by a T-Tube drainage in cholecystectomized patients after oral administration of silymarin (Legalon)." In Aktuelle Hepatologie-Symp., Koeln,November 1978, pp. 55ff. Poster (1). Hansisches Verlagskontor, Luebeck, 1979.

59. Flory, P.J., Krug, G., Lorenz, D. & Mennicke, W.H. "Biliaere elimination von silybin bei cholezystektomierten patienten nach oraler gabe von silymarin." Planta Medica,32A, 34, 1977.

60. Mennicke, W.H., Lorenz, D. & Behrendt, W. "Studies on the biliary elimination of silyÄbin in cholecystectomised patients following multiple oral administration silymarin." Naunyn-Schmiedebergs Arch. Pharmacol., 308, R29, 1979.

61. Magliulo, E., Carosi, P.G., Minoli, L. & Gorini, S. "Studies on the regenerative capacity of the liver in rats subjected to partial hepatectomy andtreated with silymarin."Arzneimittel-Forschung, 23, 161-167, 1973.

62. Sonnenbichler, J., Mattersberger, J. & Machicao, F. "Stimulierung der RNA-polymerase A und der RNA-synthese in vivo und in vitro durch ein flavonderivat." Hoppe-Seylers Z. Physiol. Chem., 357, 337, 1976.

63. Sonnenbrichler, J., Mattersberger, J. & Rosen, H. "Stimulierung der RNA-synthese in rattenleber und in isoliertenhepatozyten durch silybin, einen antihepatotoxischen wirkstoff aus silybum marianum L. Gaertn." Hoppe-Seylers Z. Physiol. Chem., 357, 1171-1180, 1976.

64. Tyutyulkova, N., et. al.,op.cit., 1983. Mandaganaro & Di Cesare, op. cit., 1977.

65. Fiebrich, G. & Koch, H. "Silymarin, an inhibitor of lipoxygenasi." Experimentia, 35, 1548, 1979.

66. Bindoli, A, Cavallini, L. & Siliprandi, N. "Inhibitory action of silymarin of lipid peroxide formation in rat liver mitochondria and microsomes." Biochem. Pharmacol., 26, 2405, 1977.

67. Vogel, G., Braatz, R. & Mengs, U. "On the nephrotoxicity of alpha-amanitin and the antagonistic effects of silymarin in rats." Agents Actions, 9, 221-226, 1979.

68. Platt, D. & Schnorr, B. "Biochemische und elektronenoptische untersuchungen zur frage der beeinflussbarkeit der aethanol-schaedigung derrattenleber durch silymarin." Arzneimittel-Forschung, 21, 1206, 1971.

69. Varkonyi, T., Maurer, R., Zoltan, O.T. & Csillik, B. "Untersuchungen ueber das durch triaethylzinnsulfat (TZS) verursachte hirnoedem bei der ratte. Arzneimittel-Forschung, 21, 148, 1971.

70. Holzgartner, H. "L'impiego della silimarina in medcina interna." Therapiewoche, 20, 698, 1968.

71. Muescher, C.H. "Silymarin bei chronischen erkrankungen der leber." Therapie der Gegenwart, 111, 1768, 1973.

72. Poser, G. "Erfahrungen mit silymarin bei der behandlung chronischer lebererkankungen." Arzneimittel-Forschung, 21, 1207-1209, 1971.

73. Hammerl, H. Pichle, O. & Studlar, M. "Uber die obiektivierung der silymarin wirkung bei lebererkrankungen." Med. Klin., 66, 1204, 1971. 74. Schadewaldt, H. "Der weg zum silymarin. Ein beitrag zur geschichte der lebertherapie." Med. Welt, 15, 902, 1969.

75. Di Palma, D. & Ciao, V. "Epatopatie croniche persistenti ed epatopatie tossiche: possibilita terapeutiche della silimarina." Cl. Terap., 94, 567, 1980.

76. Zirm, K.L. "Zur behandlung subakuter und chronischer formen der hepatitis sowie chronisch degenerativer leberkrankungen mit silymarin." Wien.Medizinischer Wochenscrift, 123, 302-305, 1973. 77. Martiis, M.D., Fontana, M., Assogna, G., D'Ottavi, R. & D'Ottavi, O. "I derivati del cardo mariano nella terapia delle epatopatie chroniche." Cl. Terap., 94(3), 283-315, 1980.

78. Floersheim, G.L., Eberhard, M., Tschumi, P. & Duckert, F. "Effects of penicillin and silyÄmarin on liver enzymes and blood clotting factors in dogs given a boiled preparation of amanita phalloides." Toxicology and Applied Pharmacology, 46, 455-462, 1978.

79. Morelli, I. "Costituenti del 'silybum marianum' e loro impiego in terapia." Boll. Chim. Farm., 117(11), 258-267, 1978.

80. Zirm, K.L., op cit., 1973.

81. Dittrich, & Hentschel, op. cit., 1970.

82. Benda, L. & Zenz, W. "Silymarin bei leberzirrhose." Wiener Medizinische Wochenschrift, 34-36, 512-516, 1973.

83. Thaler, H. "Flavonoide in der lebertherapie--ergebnisse von drei Doppelblindstudien." In Symp. "Flavonoide und Leber. Gundlagen und Bisherige Erfahrung bie der Andwendung der Flavonoide in der Lebertherapie", Frieburg/Brsg. Februar 1979. Hepatology, Rapid Literature Review V-1979, pp. 425-426. FalkFounda-

tion, Frieburg/Brsg. 1979. ì84. Salmi, H.A., Varis, K., & Siurala, M. "Treatment of alcoholic liver disease with silymarin." In Symp. "Flavonoide, etc., op.cit., pp. 429-430.
85. Saba, P., Galeone, F, Salvadorini, F., Guarguaglini, M. & Troyer, C. "Therpeutische wirkung von silymarin bei durch psychopharmaka verursachten chronischen hepatopathien." Gass. Med. Ital., 135, 236-251, 1976.
86. Benda, L., Dittrich, H., Ferenzi, P., Frank, H. & Wewelka, F. "Zur wirksamkeit von silymarin auf die ueberlebensrate von patieten mit leberzirrhose." Wein. Klin. WochenÅschrift, 92, 678-683, 1980.
87. Benda, L. & Zenz, W. "Ambulante langzeitbehandlung derleberzirrhose mit silymarin." Therapiewoche, 24, 3598-3608, 1974. 88. Fintelmann, V. & Albert, A. "Nachweis der therapeutischen Wirksamkeit von legalon bei toxischen lebererkrankungen im doppelblindversuch."Therapiewoche, 30, 5589-5594, 1980. 89. Kiesewetter, E., Leodolter, I. & Thaler, H. "Ergebnisse zweier doppelblindstudien zur wirksamkeit von silymarin bei chronischer hepatitis." Leber-Magen-Darm, 7, 318-323, 1977.
90. Plomteux, G., Albert, A. & Heusghem, C. "Hepatoprotector action of silymarin in human acute viral hepatitis." IRCS J. Med. Sci., 5, 259, 1977.
91. Schriefers, K.H. & Dietz, D. "Die beeinfulussung der leberfunktion durch legalon bei potokavalen anastomosen-operationen." Therapiewoche, 19, 1545, 1969.
92. Schopen, R.D., Lange, O.K., Panne, C. & Kirnberger, E.J. "Auf der suche nacheinem neuen therapeutischen prinzip." Med.Welt, 15, 888, 1969.
93. Schilder, M. "Silymarin in der klinischen pruefung. Ein bericht ueber 36 faellevon verschiedenen leberkrankheiten in laengsschnittuntersuchungen."Therapiewoche, 20, 3444, 1970.
94. Fintelmann, V. "Zur therapie der fettleber mit silymarin." Therapiewoche, 20, 1055, 1970.
95. Carrescia, O., Benelli, L., Saraceni, F., Braga, P.C., Cagnetta, G. & Capponi, V. "Silymarin in the prevention of hepatic damage by psychopharmacologic drugs. Experimental premises and clinical evaluation." Clin. Ter., 95, 157, 1980.
96. Hahn, G. et. al., op.cit., 1968
97. Benda & Zenz, op. cit., 1973.

Turmeric
(curcuma longa)

For The Liver, Gallbladder & Arthritis

Guaranteed Potency Constituents.

Curcumin. There are two species of curcuma with a long history of use: *curcuma longa* and *curcuma xanthorrihiza*. The first is higher in total curcumin content, the second in essential oil. The research indicates that both the curcumin and the extracted oil have similar properties, but the curcumin has the edge in terms of safety and ease of use. The oil has been observed to inflame the mucous membranes of the stomach; this safety problem, combined with difficulties in manufacture and application render the oil unsuitable for widespread consumer use.

The turmeric of choice is curcuma longa whose curcumin content can be concentrated, standardized and guaranteed at 95%.

History.

Turmeric is an herb or spice with origins in ancient southern Asia. It is now extensively cultivated in Eastern countries such as China and India, and in Western nations of the Caribbean. Turmeric provides not only flavor but color to many foods and prepared seasonings. In the West, its culinary uses far outnumber its traditional medicinal uses.

Turmeric is the primary ingredient in many varieties of curry powders and sauces. It surprises some people to learn that curry is not a single spice, nor even a uniform mixture of herbs and spices. There are as many different curries as there are people who prepare them. Other herbs often used in curry include the following: coriander, cumin, garlic, cayenne, fennel, fenugreek, anise, nutmeg, mace, cinnamon, cloves, black pepper, cardamon, ginger, and onion. Different combinations of these are used by different cultures, a different curry for vegetables than for beef, which differs from that used for chicken dishes, and so forth. The status of a cook in Asia is measured by his or her ability to combine the curry spices in just the right way to produce one of numerous anticipated effects. All must be present in a perfect balance, and careful attention must be paid to the *order* in which various spices are added. No aspect of the process is left to chance; no action is haphazard.

The selection of curry herbs over centuries of trial and error was also not the result of chance. Living in areas of the world in which foods rancidified and perished within hours, in which gastro-intestinal disease was an ever-present threat, in which vermin infested all quarters of living space, and in which food storage was a constant challenge, people constantly responded to these challenges of everyday existence by experimenting with the properties of herbs and spices. Only those that were experientially determined to be effective were incorporated into medicine and diet. Most of the effective herbs found their way into curry. The curry herbs contributed significantly to the digestion process, to the health of the liver, and to the elimination of wastes from the body.

Research in recent years has confirmed the medicinal activity of many of the curry herbs. For example, almost all of them share the following important physiological activities:

* *inhibition of platelet aggregation.* This means they prevent dangerous clotting of the blood that results when serum platelets stick together excessively. The incidence of thrombosis in countries using curry is much less than that in countries not using these spices.

* *antibiotic effects.* A single curry spice may only be effective against a very limited number of pathogens, but combinations of these spices could be effective against an incredible range of dangerous microorganisms occurring in food and the environment. Amazingly, often a particular curry will contain just the right combination of spices to eradicate just those pathogens occurring in the food for which the curry is meant to be used.

* *anti-cholesterol action.* Most of the curry herbs have been shown to prevent rises in serum cholesterol that would occur from eating fatty foods. They won't necessarily lower blood cholesterol levels directly (although some of them do, such as garlic), but when they are ingested along with the meal, they bind to cholesterolemic substances, rendering them incapable of absorption.

* *fibrinolytic activity.* This action also helps keep the blood flowing correctly. While fibrin is necessary for proper blood clotting when an injury occurs, an excess of this substance can be dangerous. Sometimes the fibrinolytic system of the body (the system that normally removes excess fibrin) malfunctions, particularly when other aspects of the body's health are being threatened. Many of the curry herbs give

the fibrinolytic system a little boost.*

The interesting thing about this constellation of effects is that they are all fairly short term in nature. These physiological actions last only as long as the herbs are in the body. But that is long enough. Your body requires the aid provided by these herbs just so long as dietary toxins, harmful fatty acids, etc., are floating around in the blood. The herbs negate the action of the harmful chemicals and boost the ability of the liver to filter them out, maintaining the health of the cells of that organ during the battle, and helping to regenerate any cells killed by toxic substances. After the digestive and assimilative war is over, the activity of the herbs ceases and the body returns to a state of rest. (The overactivity of any of these mechanisms could be just as bad as the underactivity of them — for example, blood that is in a constant state of thinning could lead to just as severe complications as blood that is in danger of clotting) This means that everybody can benefit from the frequent and proper use of various combinations of the curry herbs.

Returning to turmeric itself, a survey of the folklore literature of the world reveals that the herb has been employed in the medical systems of many nations. In China alone, turmeric is used

> "to remove blood stasis, promote and normalize energy flow in the body, and relieve pain . . . to act on the spleen and liver . . . in treating chest and rib pain, amenorrhea, abdominal mass, traumatic injuries, swelling, and carbuncles . . . treatment of hematuria (bloody urine), pain and itching of sores and ringworms, toothache, colic, flatulence, and hemorrhage".[1]

Throughout Asia, one finds the herb being used as stomachic, stimulant, carminative, hematic or styptic, to treat jaundice and other liver troubles, for irregular menstruation of all kinds, for promoting circulation, dissolving blood clots, for relieving pain, diarrhea, rheumatism, coughs, tuberculosis, and so on.

Turmeric, hardly ever used alone, is found in hundreds of different medicinal formulas. One might say it is not viewed as a primary medicinal aid, but as an important, perhaps indispensable, adjunct.

---

*This constellation of effects warrants closer attention by Western, particularly American, audiences. Our infatuation with blandness, sterility and culinary numbness has led us to the unfortunate decline in the use of these herbs. When was the last time you served curry? So what if you don't like it -- have you ever tried to make your own? There is nothing sacred about the formula you buy at the local supermarket. Try putting several of the curry herbs on your table in separate containers. Use them on your salads, poultry, soups, meats and other dishes. Discover which ones you like, and then try combining them in various ways and ratios. Personally, I find that I thoroughly dislike the flavor of coriander (which is found in almost all proprietary curries). So I leave it out. No harm done. And I have terrific curry. Use curry in your cooking as much as possible.

Method of Action.

Serious research on turmeric began in Germany, in the early 1920's. Sesquiterpenes in the essential oil of turmeric were isolated in 1926 and to them was ascribed the therapeutic activity.[2-3] Later, a team of scientists compared the effects of whole extract, the essential oil, and the water-soluble extract and found an active principle in the water extract.[4] Opinion as to the effectiveness of the pigment (curcumin) was split. Some researchers believe it contained the most important active principles; others claimed it possessed no activity whatsoever.[5-6]

Then, in 1936, an attempt was made to clarify the rather fuzzy picture that had been developing.[7] In this study curcumin was compared to whole extract and several isolated constituents. The rate of increase in secretion of bile in dogs was used as the measure of effectiveness. Applying a wide range of dosages, the scientists found that curcumin, the isolated essential oil, and p-tolymethylcarbinol (one of the constituents of the oil) were all able to increase the secretion of bile, but in differing ways, and under differing conditions. Thus, whole curcumin produced a rhythmic emptying of the gallbladder, the bile being dark and viscous, and the amount after any given contraction being small compared to the actual size of the gallbladder. The gallbladder would then immediately refill with bile and the cycle would repeat.

In contrast to curcumin, the tolymethylcarbinol produced a pure, continuous increase in the secretion of bile with no distinguishable contractions. The emptying of the gallbladder had no retrograde effect on the action of the chemical. Finally, the bile was much clearer than that produced by curcumin.

The action of the whole alcoholic extract was very similar to that of tolymethylcarbinol. However, it is to be remembered that the content of tolymethylcarbinol in the total extract is way too small to have produced the observed activity. The whole extract must have contained other substances with action similar to that of tolymethylcarbinol. The whole extract did not contain enough curcumin to produce the effects observed with the concentrate.

The above study demonstrated that turmeric contains cholagogue-type substances, with both quantitative and qualitative differences in action, which in a clinical setting, utilizing the whole herb, could account for many of the traditionally observed medicinal and physiological effects. The results of the experiment show that turmeric acts in the following ways:

* Turmeric stimulates the flow of bile; several constituents have this property.

* The increased flow of bile depends in part on the contraction of the gallbladder and in part on the increase in bile secretion;
* The stimulation of bile depends mostly on the presence of essential oil;
* The flavonoids cause the contraction of the gallbladder and thereby increase the effective emptying of this organ.

An extract of turmeric, in which the curcumin is concentrated to the extent recommended in this chapter, would possess all of the above properties.

While studies were being pursued in European, primarily German, laboratories, Asian researchers were independently validating the same properties of turmeric.[8-9] But their interest extended to liver-protective and curative principles in turmeric, and in a series of brilliant papers they reported important findings in that area. The typical experiment explored the ability of an alcohol extract to prevent the formation of lesions in the liver induced by some potent toxin, such as carbon tetrachloride, or galactosamine. The irony of these studies is, of course, that they used an alcohol extract, since alcohol is itself toxic to the liver. At any rate, the preparation provided highly significant hepato-protective activity, which led the researchers to investigate possible methods of action more closely. The results of these studies have been ambivalent; much more work is needed before we will completely understand how turmeric works. So far, what has clearly been demonstrated is that turmeric possesses anti-hepatotoxic activity on the order possessed by other liver-protective herbs such as milk thistle and licorice.[10-12]

In one of the above studies, the investigators compared the action of several turmeric constituents and their analogues, and found that only caffeic acid showed significant effect. This is an intriguing finding, since it has often been hypothesized that turmeric components somehow cleave in the body to cinnamic acid derivatives, which then show anti-hepatotoxic activity. But, in this study, it was shown that a wide variety of cinnamic acid analogues did not show significant anti-hepatotoxic effects — only caffeic acid. Since none of the most active turmeric constituents yield caffeic acid, the action of turmeric must be a result of the combined action of all curcuminoids themselves. The implication of these results is that the most effective turmeric concentrate will retain all of the major fractions of the herb. The temptation to manufacture a Guaranteed Potency alcohol extract must therefore be resisted.

Other research has helped to establish the effects of turmeric on the blood. For example, as many of the common curry herbs do, curcumin prevents large fluctuations in blood cholesterol after meals.[13]

And a very recent article reviewed research that looked specifically at the effects of curcumin on platelet aggregation inhibition and prostacyclin synthesis (anti-inflammatory principle). The herb was, of course, very effective, so much so, that the researchers recommended that it be used as a treatment of choice in patients prone to vascular thrombosis and those requiring antiarthritic therapy.[14] The authors noted the centuries old use of turmeric for these purposes in Asian medicine.

The potent anti-inflammatory activity (in the essential oil and in curcumin) of turmeric has been substantiated in other research.[15-19] Like other non-steroidal anti-inflammatory agents (such as licorice root), curcumin appears to act through some sort of adrenal mechanism (when the adrenals are removed, turmeric has no effect). Just what that mechanism is remains to be clearly determined. Licorice root acts by increasing the life of circulating steroidal substances. Perhaps turmeric operates in a similar fashion. The anti-inflammatory property compares well with many other known anti-inflammatory agents used in the treatment of arthritis.

Antibacterial and antifungal properties have been attributed to turmeric. Indeed, its effectiveness in treating cholecystitis is probably attributable to antimicrobial action.

While the basic research was being carried out, clinical information had been slowly accumulating; we turn now to a consideration of that information.

Therapeutic Research.

Liver-protection/antibiotic/anti-inflammatory effects

Except as reported in many materia medicas and pharmacopeias around the world (especially in the Orient), there has not been a great deal of clinical research published on the therapeutic action of turmeric. This is especially true of the herb's activity involving the liver: anti-hepatotoxic, antibiotic and anti-inflammatory properties. Many clinical herbal practitioners have observed these actions in their private practice, or in hospital settings, but the accounts are not even remotely scientific. For our review of the experimental or pre-clinical literature, however, I think we are justified in ascribing some large degree of reliability to clinical/quasi-anecdotal observations.

Given the similarity in action between turmeric, milk thistle, artichoke and licorice root on a pre-clinical level, involving the liver, I think we are again justified in assuming a kinship in activity among these herbs on the level of clinical practice. If that is true, it follows that turmeric will promote the health of the liver, reduce inflammation, relieve arthritic symptoms and serve as a mild antibiotic. As we will see below, the anti-inflammatory property has been effectively utilized in gallbladder disease, yet another indication that turmeric's action extends to liver disease.

Arthritis

As a note regarding turmeric's potential usefulness in the treatment of arthritis, we must acknowledge that such an effect rests entirely upon evidence concerning the herb's non-steroidal anti-inflammatory effects. Given the success that is being achieved in orthodox clinical research and practice with other non-steroidal agents, it can be assumed that there is great potential in turmeric that just needs to be exploited. Perhaps during the next few years, we will see some reports on this action begin to appear in medical journals.

We have better luck in finding clinical evidence for the effectiveness of turmeric in regard to other kinds of problems, including those reviewed below.

Cholagogue

In the normal course of research on cholagogues, animals are the primary experimental subjects. The reason for this is two-fold. First, it is infinitely easier to study this property in animals than in humans, because it usually involves some type of surgery or other invasionary tactic. Second, the results of animal studies are felt to generalize very nicely to humans. The match is not exact, however, and for that reason the occasional human study will be carried out. The one such study utilizing turmeric of which I am aware is an intriguing investigation indeed.

The study investigated the effects of a suspension of milk thistle (*carduus marianus*), celandine (*chelidonium majus*) and turmeric on choleretic activity in 28 healthy patients.[20] The cholagogue activity of celandine and milk thistle are known to be very limited.[21-23] Now, even a very good cholagogue will only raise the production of bile in healthy humans by about 25-49% (can be much greater in experimental animals). In this case, however, the volume of bile rose by an incredible 369% compared to baseline levels. A similar extraordinary rise in the secretion of bilirubin was observed (285%). These results indicate that the interactions among the principles of cholagogues are not simply additive, nor even clearly multiplicative, but involve a synergistic mechanism that will require much more research before it is understood.

Gallbladder disease

A number of studies have shown that curcumin both protects the gall bladder against disease and is a good treatment for such disease. The successful treatment of gallstones (cholelithiasis), acute and chronic inflammation of the gall bladder (cholecystitis), and inflammation of the bile duct (cholangitis) have been reported.[24] The effectiveness of turmeric in the latter two conditions is probably due to its anti-inflammatory and antibacterial properties. And, as mentioned above, the action of turmeric in disorders of the gall bladder is probably a very good indication that the herb has similar effects on the equivalent and similar conditions in the liver.

Therapeutic Action.

Digestion/cholagogue

The centuries old use of turmeric as a stomachic and carminative, as well as its routine inclusion in curry, in countries covering three quarters of the world's surface, are sufficient evidence to validate its purported beneficial effects on the digestive processes.

There is a tendency in the medical world to downplay the role of the gall bladder and of bile in digestion. That may be why the gall bladder is so often surgically removed when gallstones are present. At any rate, the statement is often heard that people who have had their gallbladder removed lead perfectly normal lives thereafter, without hardly noticing anything different.

We don't want to argue that point here (though it is arguable), but we do want to emphasize the fact that though the absence of the gallbladder may be tolerable, the *presence* of a healthy, functioning gallbladder (and bile duct) can contribute a great deal to increased digestive effectiveness which directly decreases the chances of arteriosclerosis, irritable bowel syndrome, hypertension, heart disease, stroke, and so forth. After all, if you die of a stroke who is going to blame it on that gallbladder operation you had five years ago? Likewise, if you live to be 100 who's going to say it is because you still have a healthy gallbladder? Cause and effect in this area are extremely tenuous. So why take chances?

In a similar vein, the choleretic effects of turmeric may be intimately related to its liver-protective properties. Everything more or less acts together in this area of functional anatomy. I think one's chances of a healthy vigorous life are greatly improved by making certain everything stays intact and functioning.

Since we have devoted so much space toward establishing turmeric as a good cholagogue, we need to clarify just when, and when not, to use a cholagogue. Use it under the following conditions:

for long term maintenance of dyskinesia of the bile duct; for stimulating normal reflexive contractions of this organ in order to deliver bile to the small intestine.

for disorders caused by insufficient or congested bile, such as intractable biliary constipation, jaundice and mild hepatitis.

for the treatment of autonomic functional disorders in the epigastric area; for symptoms of indigestion to aid in the digestion of fat-soluble substances, particularly certain vitamins and acid foods.

for help in cleansing the liver and in helping it filter wastes and toxins from the body.

for gallstones, unless they are lodged in the bile duct and causing a great deal of pain.

Cholagogues are not indicated and should be avoided under the following conditions:

painful gallstones; the increased contractile activity could further constrict the bile duct leading to incredibly intense pain.

acute bilious colic.

obstructive jaundice; the same reservations apply here as with painful gallstones.

Acute cholecystitis (inflammation of the gallbladder) unless gallstones have been ruled out; cholecystitis can be caused by infection, but you should determine the cause before using a cholagogue.

Acute viral hepatitis, although herbs such as turmeric may be used in sub-cholagogue doses, since they contribute so greatly to repair of the liver and destruction of the infectious agents; nevertheless, even in the case of turmeric, it may be well to wait until the acute phase is past. Best advice: Proceed with caution.

Extremely toxic liver disorders; a cholagogue may be too stressful for a liver that is damaged to this extent; but again, this must be weighed against the potential benefit to be derived from the liver-protecting properties of the particular herb. Personally, I wouldn't hesitate to use mild doses of turmeric, avoiding the combination of celandine, turmeric and milk thistle discussed earlier.

Weight loss

Another aspect of turmeric use is its potential contribution to certain kinds of weight loss programs. Because it aids in the breakdown (catabolism) and metabolism of fats in the liver, turmeric contributes important factors to weight reduction procedures. It has been reported that the Caraka Samhits of ancient India (3,000 B.C.) recommended a certain herbal preparation, that included turmeric, for the treatment of obesity .[25] You say you are not convinced? Well, hey, give it a try. . . .

Gallbladder disorders

Whereas the literature supporting the use of turmeric for liver disorders is lacking, there is at least some good evidence for the use of this herb in the treatment of various gallbladder problems. It can safely be recommended as a treatment of choice for gallstones (cholelithiasis) that are not presently painfully lodged in the bile duct, acute and chronic inflammation of the gall bladder (cholecystitis), and inflammation of the bile duct (cholangitis). The reason you wouldn't use turmeric to get rid of stuck and painful gallstones is that the cholekinetic (bile duct stimulant) property of curcumin could cause contractions of the duct in the immediate vicinity of the stones — that could be a very painful experience. Before treating yourself for disorders of the gallbladder, you would wisely obtain medical confirmation of your problem.

Snake bite

While we bemoan the paucity of good clinical data on many of the properties of turmeric that offer applications approaching worldwide significance, we discover a great quantity of research detailing the antidotal effects of *curcuma* species on Thai cobra bites. I guess such research is of extreme importance to the Thais. At any rate, the *antidotal* publications on turmeric and snake bite are far more numerous than the *anecdotal* publications on liver disorders.

In Thai folk medicine, a tea made from *curcuma* species is given orally to victims of the bite of *Naja naja siamensis*, and is said to produce recovery from this normally very lethal envenomization. Given intravenously to mice and dogs, the tea seems to be a very effective antidote.[26-27] On the basis of the findings of several related studies, the mechanism of action appears to be one of direct inactivation; the exact manner in which this takes place is unknown.[28-29]

One of the interesting by-products of this research has been the discovery of proteolytic (protein-digestive) activity in turmeric.[30] A pair of scientists had reasoned that the inactivation of the cobra venom might be the result of some proteolytic activity in the turmeric extract since the venom is itself a polypeptide (protein). Consequently, they first attempted to find a protein-digesting moiety in the extract — and succeeded. Unfortunately for their research, this fraction turned out to

136

be inactive against the venom. But fortunately for us, we now know of two distinct ways by which turmeric aids in the digestive process; *indirectly*, through the circuitous route of bile production, storage and secretion, and through a *direct* action on dietary proteins.

Route of Administration.

Turmeric is almost always administered orally. A case could be made for intravenous administration under extremely severe circumstances, but there is certainly no reason for taking such measures 99% of the time.

Some medicinal value is bound to accrue from turmeric sprinkled liberally on all kinds of foods, and included in curry. But medicinal value is better assured when Guaranteed Potency turmeric is taken internally in capsules. In addition, this form of turmeric makes an excellent addition to many herbal formulas geared to the kind of problems discussed in this chapter.

Dosage.

Taken by itself, one 300 mg. capsule at each meal (or at two of three meals) per day is sufficient. Combined with other herbs, anywhere from 50 mg. to 150 mg. is sufficient.

Toxicity.

No toxicity has been observed at recommended dosages. In exceedingly high amounts, it has been observed to inflame the mucous linings of the stomach. Since this reaction is similar to that of cayenne on 'innocent' tissue, it is possible that the stomach lining would adapt to the presence of turmeric over time, eventually exhibiting no inflammation at all to even very high doses.

References.

1. Leung, A.Y. Chinese Herbal Remedies, Universe Books, New York, 1984, p. 164.
2. Guttenberg, A. Klin. Wschr., , 1926, p. 1998. (cited in Robbers, H. below.
3. Dieterle, H. & Kaiser, P. In Arch. Pharmazie Ber., dtsch Ges., 270, 413, 1932.
4. Kalk, H. & Nissen, K. "Untersuchungen ueber die wirkung der cucuma (Temoe Lawak) auf die funktion der leber und der gallenwege." Dtsch. Med. Wschr., 36, 1613, 1931. And Kalk, H. & Nissen, K. Dtsch. Med. Wschr., 44, 1932. (cited in Robbeers, H., below.)
5. Franquelo, E. Muench. Med. Woschr., 1933, p. 524. (cited in Robbers, H., below.)
6. Grabe, F. Naunyn Schmiederbergs Arc. Pharm., 176, 673, 1934.
7. Robbers, H. "Ueber den wirkungsmechanismus der einzelnen curcumabestandteile

auf die gallensekretion." Archiv fuer Experimental. Path. und Pharmacol., 181, 328-334, 1936.

8. Ramprasad, C. & Sirsi, M. J. of Scientific Indian Medical Research, Sect C, 15, 262, 1956.

9. Ramprasad, C. & Sirsi, M. J. of Scientific Indian Medical Research, Sect C, 16, 108, 1957.

10. Kiso, Y., Suzuki, Y., Konno, C. Hikino, H. Hashimoto, I. & Yagi, Y. "Application of carbon tetrachloride-induced liver lesion in mice for screening of liver protective crude drugs. Shoyakugaku Zasshi, 36, 238-244, 1982.

11. Kiso, Y., Tohkin, M. & Hikino, H. "Assay method for antihepatotoxic activity using carbon tetrachloride-induced cytotoxicity in primary cultured hepatocytes." Planta Medica, 49, 222-225, 1983.

12. Kiso, Y. Suzuki, Y., Watanabe, N., Oshima, Y. & Hikino, H. "Antihepatotoxic principles of curcuma longa rhizomes." Planta Medica, 49, 185-187, 1983.

13. Leung, A. Encyclopedia of Common Natural Ingredients in Food, Drugs, and Cosmetics, John Wiley & Sons, New York City, New York, 1980.

14. Srivastava, R. Puri, V., Srimal, R.C. & Dhawan, R.N. "Effect of curcumin on platelet aggregation and vascular prostacyclin synth." Arzneimittel-Forschung, 36(4), 715-717, 1986.

15. Srimal, R.C. & Dhaman, B.N. "Pharmacology of diferuloyl methane (curcumin), a non-steroidal anti-inflammatory agent." J. Pharm. Pharmacol., 25, 447-452, 1973.

16. Mukhodapadhyay, A., Basu, N., Ghatak, N. & Gujral, P. "Anti-inflammatory and irritant activities of curcumin analogues in rats." Agents Actions, 12, 508-515, 1982.

17. Chandra, D. & Gupta, S. "Anti-inflammatory and anti- arthritic activity of volatile oil of curcuman longa (Haldi). Indian Journal of Medical Research, 60, 138-142, 1972.

18. Arora, R., Basu, N. Kapoor, V. & Jain, A. "Anti-inflammatory studies on curcuma longa (turmeric). Indian Journal of Medical Research, 56, 1289-1295, 1971.

19. Ghatak, N. & Basu, N. "Sodium curcuminate as an effective anti-inflammatory agent." Indian Journal of Experimental Biology, 10, 235-236, 1972.

20. Bauman, J. Ch., Heintze, H. & Muth, H.W. "Klinisch-experimentelle untersuchungen der gallen-, magen-, und pankreassekretion unter den phytocholagogen wirkstoffen einer carduus marianus-chelidonium- curcuma-suspension." Arzneimittel- Forschung, 26, 98, 1971.

21. Goetz, H.G., op. cit.

22. Zaterka, S. & Grossman, M.I. "The effect of gastrin and histamine on secretion of bile." Gastroenterology, 50, 500, 1966. 23. Maiwald, L. "Pflanzliche cholagoga." Zhurnal der Allgemein Medizin, 59, 304-308, 1983.

24. Luckner, et. al., op. cit.

25. Trivedi, V.P. & Mann, A.S. "Vegetable drugs regulating fat metabolism in Caraka (Lekhaniya dravyas)." Quarterly Journal of Crude Drug Research, 12(4), 1988-1999, 1972.

26. Tejasen, P. Chantaratham, A. & Kanjanapothi, D. "The antagonistic effect of a medicinal plant (curcuma sp., zingiberaceae) to Thailand cobra venom (Naja naja siamensis). Part I." Chaing Mai Med. Bull., 8, 165, 1969.

27. Tejasen, P. & Sunyapridakul, L. "Experimental studies of the effect of an aqueous extract of Wan Ngu (curcuma sp., zingibeaceae) on cobra envenomization." Chiang Mai Med. Bull., 9, 56, 1970.

28. Cherdchu, C. Srisukawat, K. & Ratanabanangkoon, K. "Cobra neurotoxin inhibiting activity found in the extract of curcuma sp. (zingiberaceae)." Journal of the Medical Association of Thailand, 61, 544, 1978.

29. Chantaratham, A. & Tejasen, P. "Studies of the antagonistic effect of Wan Ngu (curcuma sp., Zingiberaceae) on the action of Thailand cobra venom (Naja naja siamensis) at the neuromuscular junction." Chiang Mai Med. Bull., 9, 73, 1970.

30. Cherdchu, C. & Karlsson, E. "Proteolytic-independent cobra neurotoxin inhibiting activity of curcuma sp. (zingiberaceae)." Southeast Asian Journal of Tropical Medicine and Public Health, 14(2), 176, 1983.

III. Flavonoids

The reader will have noticed that several of the Guaranteed Potency constituents in the foregoing chapters were examples of flavonoids. Next to chlorophyll and the carotenoids, the flavonoids are the most prevalent pigments in the plant kingdom. They are also some of the most widespread biologically active substances in plants. Some of the most often encountered flavonoids are quercitin, catechin, rutin, anthocyanidin, khellin, asculetine, luteolin, apiin, kampferol, astragelin, and hesperidin. Together, the flavonoids are called vitamin P, even though their action differs rather significantly from that of other vitamins.

This short section is included to give the reader an overview of the wide-ranging activity of these substances. It is true that several have been highlighted in this book, but there are undoubtedly others present in the herbs discussed that contribute, to one degree or another, to the overall medicinal value.

The following is a list of the physiological properties of flavonoids that have been verified in basic research. Even though such a list suggests that the effects are individual and descrete, this is not the case. Rather, there is a great deal of interaction and interdependency. For example, the anti-inflammatory property is intrinsically related to the anti-hyaluronidase, membrane stabilizing and anti-oxidant effects and probably others. This list, then, is at once a detailed presentation of physiological properties and an oversimplification of total action.

1. *Anti-oxidant.* The particular mechanisms of action involved here are still not entirely clear, but it is no longer questioned that the flavonoids possess a considerable anti-oxidant effect. Quercetin and catechin are particularly powerful anti-oxidants. The anti-oxidant effect prevents the formation free radicals and inflammatory leukotrienes. Flavonoids are also very good at inhibiting the oxidation of ascorbic acid, thereby possibly greatly potentiating its action.

2. *Anti-hyaluronidase.* Refer to the chapter on echinacea for a detailed discussion of this property. Catechin, rutin, quercetin and hesperidin all possess this action to a considerable degree.

3. The ability to increase the circulation time of corticosteroids, in a way similar to the ginsenosides from ginseng.

4. The ability to lower blood sugar level by influencing the metabolism of carbohydrates. A good benefit for diabetics.

5. Capillary-permeability -stabilizing. This ability to prevent capillary walls from becoming permeable and hence less resistant to leakage gave flavonoids the name vitamin P (permeability). This property is somehow tied to that of histamine. In experimental settings, flavonoids such as catechin and quercetin are able to prevent allergic reactions (and anaphylactic shock) induced by histamine. The mechanism of action appears to be inhibition of the release of histamine from mast cells and basophils.

6. *Anti-inflammatory.*

7. *Anti-leukotrienes.* Flavonoids may inhibit leukotriene formation both through an anti-oxidant property and by interrupting the synthetic pathway directly.

8. *Immunostimulating.* Stimulates antibody production, T-cell formation and lymphocyte transformation. Particularly true of catechin.

9. *Anti-hepatotoxic.* Catechin and other flavonoids inhibit the activity of endotoxins (potent liver-damaging chemicals produced by bacteria) when the RES (reticulo-endothelial system) and the immune-response systems break down and are no longer able to destroy these chemicals naturally.

10. *Hypotensive.*

11. *Anti-tumor.* May depend on its anti-leukotrienes, anti-oxidant, and antibiotic properties. Quercetin is particularly active.

12. *Connective tissue regulating.* Flavonoids, especially catechin, seem to be capable of promoting the formation and stablization of connective tissue under normal conditions, but to inhibit its overproduction in post operative situations. Catechin is also very effective in improving the outlook for *osteogenesis imperfecta* patients — who normally suffer from considerable bone fragility — by stabilizing collagen-based connective tissues surrounding the bones.

13. *Sedative.*

14. Ability to increase the red blood cell count in anemia.

15. *Cardiac regulating* properties, that probably arise from the ability of flavonoids to increase the flow of blood through the coronary vessels.

16. A very weak *estrogenic* effect.

17. *Antibacterial/Antiviral.*

18. *Enzyme-regulating.*

19. *Anti-spasmodic.* Very strong and thoroughly researched effect.

20. *Diuretic.*

21. *Cholagogue.*

22. *Hemostatic, styptic.*

Part Two: The Combinations

I. Introduction & Rationale

Herbs have been combined for as long as herbs have been used. Herbal practitioners of every age, in every land, have discovered that combinations of herbs usually, but not always, exert a more subtle, well-balanced, and reliable effect on the physiology of the body than single herbs.

From a scientific point of view, herbal combinations are a nightmare. Even a cursory inspection of the art of combining herbs reveals the necessity for performing thousands of experiments in any effort to untangle the myriad interactions involved. Some European scientists have spent their entire careers just trying to understand the interactions among three or four simple herbs. A concerted effort on the part of the entire scientific community would still take hundreds of years to complete.

And so in the absence of scientific data on herbal combinations, we are left to our own devices. We must rely on our own common sense, but must be guided by valid principles. Often our combinations will depend on nothing more than what feels good. But if our intuition is on target, that might be a valid method. Sometimes I look at combinations and they just don't seem right; I can't exactly spell out my objections — I just know something is not right. Of course, the more we do know about herbs, the better judgement we will have. And sometimes the critical factor is not *how* our knowledge is obtained, but how capable we are of evaluating and judging it. If I were to pit my laboratory knowledge against the hands-on knowledge of a competent herbalist, I would lose every time. The pivotal word here is "competent." I think that sometimes my objectivity puts me in a better position than that of herbalists who let such criteria as ego-involvement, astrological expectation, and metaphysical mumbo jumbo cloud their judgements. But even that is not absolute.

Combining herbs is thus, at least for now, an art, a skilled art to be sure, but one that is subject to individual preferences. The combining of Guaranteed Potency herbs may raise the level of the art a notch or two. At least the use of such products will eliminate one source of variability in observed medicinal outcomes. Personal variables will remain the same as always, but variability in plant materials will be eliminated. Variability in concentration among the various combined herbs will remain, but we should be able to get a better grasp of the meaning of this variableness as time goes on.

Therefore, combinations of Guaranteed Potency herbs are realistically the next generation in herbal medicine (someday I may get around to figuring out which generation that is). They can be combined with each other, with other non-guaranteed powdered herbs, with vitamins, minerals, isolates, and so forth.

Combination or Single?

But when should you choose a combination and when should you choose the single herb? Why should you use a combination built around milk thistle instead of using milk thistle by itself? The answer to these questions depends upon several factors, not the least of which is simply personal preference. Some people prefer the straightforward approach, the simpler the better; combinations, blends, formulas — these are too confusing. As long as you are only interested in the main, predominant effects of the herb, the straightforward approach is alright. I often use ginger root all by itself, but I seldom use cascara sagrada by itself. What's the difference? They are both effective therapeutic agents for the gastro-intestinal tract, and they can both be relied upon to produce certain results. So why would I treat them any different in practice? The reason is that the action of cascara actually *improves* when it is combined with other herbs. *Improvement* does not necessarily mean *augmentation*. The effects of cascara, for example, due not usually need to be augmented. Improvement can also involve subtle changes that make the herb more *pleasant* in action, more *flavorful*, more easily *digested* and *assimilated*; it can involve an *extension in activity* into other areas, an *elimination of side effects*, and so forth. The more we understand about the actions of herbs the better able we are to *complement* the action of one with a group of others.

So one time you would choose a combination over a single herb is when you recognize that certain advantages provided by the blend correspond with your own needs. Singles are often a good starting place for herbal neophytes, but most herb users normally begin to include more and more combinations.

what kind of language is this

II. The Guaranteed Potency Combinations

Milk Thistle Combination

Ingredients

> Milk thistle (*Silybum marianum*)
> Turmeric (*Curcuma longa*)
> Pale Catechu (*Uncaria gambir*)

Rationale

The primary purpose of this combination is to provide nutritive and therapeutic support for the liver, both in terms of protection and in terms of restoration, or healing. The mild cholagogue properties of milk thistle are augmented by turmeric, and the mild liver-protecting properties of turmeric are augmented by milk thistle. While milk thistle unquestionably has the most potent anti-hepatotoxic properties, turmeric contributes important anti-inflammatory and antibiotic effects that complement those of milk thistle. Dandelion root, while not a Guaranteed Potency herb, is nonetheless one of the safest and most effective liver tonics in the plant kingdom. It not only provides excellent therapeutic support, but is also highly nutritive. Among its medicinal properties are these: cholagogue; liver-protective; effective treatment for hepatitis, jaundice, gallstones, bile duct inflammation and dyskinesia, and indigestion. For a more complete review of the medicinal properties of dandelion root the reader is referred to my earlier work, The Scientific Validation of Herbal Medicine.

Dandelion also provides a broad range of nutrients from which the body can draw for regeneration and maintenance; sometimes, in our zealousness to medicate, we overlook the importance of such support. Since this combination is designed to provide total care for the liver, the presence of dandelion root is insurance that that goal is reached.

The beneficial and complementary effects of these three products on virtually every aspect of the digestive system make this combination a truly superior product. When the digestive system needs a boost, particularly in the presence of indigestion, flatulence, heartburn, etc., the blend should be a very powerful aid.

Use

For the prevention and treatment of liver disorders, including toxic-metabolic disease, acute viral hepatitis, chronic-persistent hepatitis, chronic-aggressive hepatitis, cirrhosis, fatty degeneration and others.

For the support of gallbladder function, including the secretion of bile by the liver, the storage of bile in the gallbladder, the contraction of the gallbladder proper, and the contraction of the bile duct.

For the improvement of all digestive processes. To promote the health of liver, gallbladder, spleen, kidneys, stomach, intestines. To promote the health of the blood that supplies all of these important organs.

Doses

Routine maintenance and prevention: 1 capsule with meals.
Acute and chronic conditions: 1-3 capsules with meals.

Toxicity and Contraindications

These herbs are without toxicity. However, care must be taken when using this combination in the presence of extremely toxic liver disorders, as the cholagogue action may be cause some discomfort. In such conditions, for a pure and simple curative effect on the disorder, use milk thistle as a single herb.

Ginkgo Biloba Combination

Ingredients

Ginkgo (*Ginkgo biloba*)
Bilberry (*Vaccinum myrtillus*)
Centella (*Centella asiatica*)
Ginger (*Zingiber officinale*)

Ginger root is used as a base for the other herbs and acts as an activator in the gastro-intestinal tract.

Rationale

Much is gained by combining the properties of ginkgo, bilberry and centella. The emphasis in this combination is on the cerebral actions of ginkgo (Alzheimer's disease, memory loss, dementia, etc.), but certainly it is also meant to support, both structurally and functionally, the many other profound effects of ginkgo on the vascularity and neuro-physiology of the body. The effect of bilberry on the permeability and, hence, the integrity of the walls of vessels and capillaries is even more direct and significant than that of ginkgo. Hence, the presence of bilberry both supports and extends the action of ginkgo on the vascularity. Centella contributes its well-known neural tonic and connective tissue stabilizing properties, as well as its distinct anti-sclerotic property. This latter property nicely complements the actions of bilberry and ginkgo. Whereas the latter two herbs have a pronounced tendency to reduce congestion and hardening of the arteries, experimental trials indicates that centella may be even more effective. Also, the unique and specific action of centella on phlebitis appears to be missing from the constellation of effects attributed to ginkgo. The combination of these three herbs should make a substantial contribution to the herbal armamentarium.

Use

For the prevention and treatment of a wide variety of neuro-vascular disorders, including arterial and venous, peripheral and central, functional and structural disorders. Examples: peripheral arterial and venous insufficiency (manifested by phlebitis, intermittent claudication, cold and pallor in toes, circulatory disorders of the skin — including ulcers, bed sores, eczema — chronic arterial obliteration, pain, cramps, heaviness in legs, hemorrhoids, etc.); cerebral circulatory insufficiency (manifested by dementia, memory loss, visual disorders, headache, etc.); sclerosis, both arterial and venous.

For the regulation of vessel tone, both peripherally and centrally, by being simultaneously anti-spasmodic and tonic, and by toning capillary walls, reducing fragility and hyperpermeability.

For the support of the body's tissue repair processes, by insuring the integrity of blood flow toward damaged or inflamed areas, and the efficient removal of wastes and toxins.

For the prevention and treatment of dementia, Alzheimer's disease, and other disorders of the central nervous system with neural and/or vascular and/or endocrine components. For the improvement or restitution of alertness, memory, ability to concentrate, cognitive function and mental capacity. To remove depression and anxiety. To delay deterioration and restore function in all supportive physiological substrates.

For prevention and treatment of vascular disturbances of the inner ear, including vertigo, tinnitus, headache, partial deafness.

For the internal treatment of hemorrhoids, by decreasing congestion and bleeding.

For the prevention and treatment of physiological damage due to the presence of free radicals: including cancer, diabetes, blindness and atherosclerosis.

For the prevention of diabetic complications including neuropathy, angiopathy, and hypertension.

Doses

Routine maintenance and prevention: 1-2 capsules per day.
Acute and chronic conditions: 2-5 capsules per day.

Toxicity and Contraindications

All of the ingredients in the this blend are well-tolerated, and have exhibited no toxic effects or allergic reactions in doses many times greater than those recommended here.

No contraindications are known.

Centella Combination

Ingredients

Centella (*Centella asiatica*)
Bilberry (*Vaccinum myrtillus*)
Butcher's Broom (*Ruscus aculeatus*)
Ginger root (*Zingiber officinale*)

Ginger root is used as a base for the other herbs and acts as an activator in the gastro-intestinal tract.

146

Rationale

This combination is primarily designed to be used in the prevention and treatment of circulatory disorders, especially in the areas of proctology (hemorrhoids), phlebology (varicose veins, chilblains, etc.), ophthalmology (retinopathy, glaucoma) and gynecology (menstrual problems, milk legs, etc.). Each of the three main herbs contributes, in its own way, complementary actions on the arteries and veins and the connective tissues that surround and support them. The effects are manifested in virtually every part of the body, from the eyes to the rectum, from the outer skin tissues to the inner cells of the brain and heart.

Use

For the prevention and treatment of proctological problems, including hemorrhoids, proctitis, pruritus, anal fissures, and related conditions.

For the prevention and treatment of disorders of the veins and arteries, including varicose veins, chilblains, "heavy" legs, venous circulatory disorders, edema, ulcers, thrombosis, insufficiency, hypertension, diabetic complications, phlebitis, arteriosclerosis, purpuras, hematuria, bleeding gums, etc.

For the prevention and treatment of disorders of the eyes, including diabetic glaucoma, diabetic retinopathy, retinal hemorrhages, eye strain, myopia, cataracts, etc.

For the prevention and treatment of gynecological problems, including menstrual problems, cramps, varicose veins of pregnancy (milk legs), and delivery-related problems (lesions, ulcers, etc).

Doses

Routine maintenance and prevention: 1-2 capsules per day.
Acute conditions: 2-4 capsules per day.
Chronic conditions: 1-4 capsules per day.

Toxicity and Contraindications

None.

Bilberry Combination

Ingredients

>   Bilberry (*Vaccinum myrtillus*)
>   Quercetin
>   Beta-carotene
>   Vitamins: A, E, B6
>   Trace Elements: GTF Chromium, Zinc, Selenium
>   Amino Acids: L-cysteine, L-glutamine, L-glycine,Taurine

Quercetin is probably the leading flavonoid. It contributes immensely to this blend. First it complements the anti-diabetic property of bilberry by inhibiting the enzyme aldose reductase, which is believed responsible for promoting the formation of diabetic cataracts, neuropathy and retinopathy, and by stimulating the secretion of insulin. In addition, its anti-oxidant properties inhibit the toxic effects of free radicals on the pancreatic beta cells (a good review of these properties is provided by Pizzorno & Murray in their A Textbook of Natural Medicine). Quercetin also augments the capillary stabilization properties of bilberry.

Beta-carotene, a naturally occurring precursor of vitamin A, has many important biological properties. Two of those are very important to the effectiveness of a bilberry combination. First, it is converted easily and directly into retinol and stored in the liver for use in sustaining normal vision capabilities. Second, it is one the best anti-oxidants known, thus augmenting not only the action of bilberry but complementing that of quercetin as well.

Rationale

Research over the past twenty years has shown that a major therapeutic treatment for eye disorders can be structured around bilberry. The physiological properties of bilberry are profound, but those properties can be strengthened, augmented, complemented, and extended by the addition of certain naturally occurring nutrients. Chief among these are the flavonoid quercetin, and beta-carotene. Also of importance in the health of the eyes are a handful of other essential nutrients (as listed above). Proprietary bilberry-containing medicines, available in Europe, normally contain several of the supporting nutrients.

Use

For the prevention and treatment of eye disorders, including diabetic neuropathy, cataract, night blindness, myopia, blood purpuras. For enlarging the range of vision and improving visual acuity.

For the prevention and treatment of varices and other arterial and venous troubles, including brain circulatory disturbances.

In diabetes, as a vasodilator, hypotensor, and protector of capillary walls.

For toning capillary walls, by reducing capillary fragility and hyperpermeability, thereby reducing the spread of wastes and toxins through the tissues.

Doses

Routine maintenance and prevention: 1-2 capsules per day.
Acute and chronic conditions: 1-3 capsules per day.

Toxicity and Contraindications

All of the ingredients in this blend are safe if used as recommended. The three main ingredients, bilberry, quercetin and beta-carotene, are well tolerated even in amounts greatly exceeding those recommended here. The remaining ingredients are present in small enough amounts to also present no problem, even if the daily dose recommendation is greatly exceeded.

No contraindications are known for these products. Diabetics should be under a physician's supervision.

III. Guaranteed Potency Herbs
(To Augment Traditional Blends)

One of the most important uses for Guaranteed Potency Herbs is to augment the effectiveness of regular encapsulated herbal blends. It would be a big mistake to get rid of the regular blends at this time. Decades of research will be required to ascertain the feasibility of standardizing even the most important constituents of the most common herbs. And that is not enough; one must still match biological activity to constituent or groups of constituents, observe and record important interactions, and do all the necessary toxicity studies. And when all of that is done, there is still no guarantee it will yield a product worth the expense of standardizing — to producer or to customer.

Currently, the best course of action is to keep and use our regular herbs and herbal blends. In fact, with the addition of just the few Guaranteed Potency herbs introduced in this book, the usefulness of regular herbal blends can be *increased* substantially; **therefore, the future should see a stimulated interest in and use of regular herbal blends.**

To kick things off, I will show how one might go about combining the use of the products discussed in this book with the blends presented in The Scientific Validation of Herbal Medicine and Proven Herbal Blends (those books are only a couple of years old, and are already in need of up-dating, it appears).

Chapter Titles/Conditions	Supplment With
Arthritis	butcher's broom, ginseng, turmeric
High Blood Pressure	ginseng
Blood Purification & Detoxification	echinacea, milk thistle
Blood Sugar, Low	ginseng
Bone-Flesh-Cartilage	centella
Cholesterol Regulation	milk thistle, turmeric
Circulation	bilberry, butcher's broom, centella, ginkgo, ginseng
Detoxify/Nurture	echinacea
Diabetes	bilberry, butcher's broom,

	centella, ginkgo, ginseng
Digestion	milk thistle, turmeric
Diuretic	-----------------------
Environmental Pollution	ginseng
Eyes	bilberry
Fatigue	ginseng, centella, ginkgo
Female Tonic	centella, ginseng
Fevers & Infections	echinacea, ginseng
Hayfever & Allergy	echinacea
Heart Tonic	bilberry, butcher's broom, centella, ginkgo, ginseng
Hemorrhoids/Astringent	bilberry, butcher's broom, centella, ginkgo
Infertility	ginseng
Influenza	echinacea
Insomnia	ginseng
Laxative	milk thistle
Liver Disorders	milk thistle, turmeric
Menstruation	-----------------------
Mental Alertness/Senility	centella, ginkgo, ginseng
Nausea	turmeric
Nerves & Glands	bilberry, centella, ginkgo, ginseng
Nervous Tension	ginkgo, ginseng
Pain Relief	-----------------------
Parasites & Worms	-----------------------
Prostate Problems	ginseng, turmeric
Respiratory Ailments	echinacea
Skin Disorders	bilberry, butcher's broom, centella, echinacea
Stomach/Intestinal Problems	milk thistle, turmeric
Thyroid	ginseng
Various Yeast Infections	echinacea, turmeric
Weight Loss	turmeric
Whole Body Tonic	centella, ginseng

Index

153

depression, 76, 81, 102, 146
detoxification, 120
dexamethasone, 97
diabetes, 19, 21, 66, 102, 146ff
diabetic angiopathy, 70, 78, 146, 148
diabetic neuropathy, 146, 148
digestion, 98f, 129, 134, 144
digestive disorders, 109f
diptheria, 46, 57
discrimination, 91
diuretic, 109, 140
DNA, 89, 95, 98, 101
dopamine, 67f, 81
drug abuse, 121
dyskinesia, 143
dyspepsia, 109
echinacea (*echinacea angustifolia*), 45ff, 151
echinacosides, 45ff
eclectic physicians, 46f, 57f
eczema, 36, 145
edema, 28f, 65f, 147
EEG, 89
endoplasmic reticulum, 95
endurance, 101
entero-hepatic circuit, 117f
enzymes, 50
eosinophils, 50
ephedra, 11
ephedrine, 11
epinephrine, 68, 81
episiotomy, 37
erysipelas, 38, 42, 46
estrogenic, 90, 140
exhaustion, 102
eye strain and disease, 15ff, 21ff, 147ff
5-HT, 54 (*see also serotonin*)
fatigue, 102
fertility, 101
fever, 33, 46
fibrin, 49, 128
fibrinolytic, 128
flatulence, 129, 144
flavoglycosides, 63ff
flavonoids, 12, 63ff, 80, 108ff, 117, 130, 139f, 148

food, rancidification of, 128
food poisoning, 115
free radical inhibition, 66, 76, 79f, 116f, 146
freeze-dried herbs, 8
Frog virus 3 (FV3), 114f
galactosamine, 116, 131
gallbladder, 109, 130f, 134, 144
gallbladder disease, 134, 136
gallstones, 109f, 134f, 143
gamma-globulins, 51, 94f
gastritis, 98
geriatrics, 74ff
giardia, 12
ginger root, 7-8, 144ff
ginseng (*panax ginseng*), 87ff, 151
Ginseng Abuse Syndrome, 104ff
ginsenosides, 87ff
ginkgo (*ginkgo biloba*), 63ff, 144f, 151
glaucoma, 20, 21, 147
glucoronic acid, 117
glucose-6-phosphatase, 16
glycosides, 47
goldenseal, 12
granules, 50
ground substance, 56
gums, bleeding, 147
gynecology, 29, 36f, 147
headache, 33, 71f, 76, 78, 102, 145f
hearing loss, 72, 80
heart, 17, 66, 147
heartburn, 143
heart disease, 102, 134
heaviness in legs, 28f, 40, 145
hematuria, 20, 21, 129, 147
hemeralopia, 18
hemorrhage, 129
hemorrhoids, 26ff, 73f, 81, 145ff
hemorrhoidal knots, 29
hemostatic, 140
hepatitis, 109, 115, 118, 119ff, 135, 143f
hepatoprotection, 112ff, 131ff, 134, 143
herb industry, 8
herpes, 55

monocytes, 50
mucopolysaccharides, 49
mucous membranes, 127
myopia, 15ff, 147
nearsightedness, 15ff
necrosis, 114
nerve tonic, 33
nervousness, 102
neurological disorders, 76
neurosis, 102
neurotransmitters, 67ff, 81
neurovascular disorders, 145
neutrophils, 46, 50
night blindness, 15ff
nocturnal cramps, 40
noradrenergic, 68f
norepinephrine, 68, 81
nutritive, 143
nyctalopia, 15ff
obesity, 39
obstetrics, 20
ophthalmology, 29, 147
opsin, 15f
osteogenesis imperfecta, 140
oxygen, 79, 117f
oxygen scavengers, 66, 80
parasympathetic, 92
Parkinson's disease, 71
peripheral arteriopathy, 71, 77
peripheral vascular insufficiency, 69
peritonitis, 110
periwinkle, 12
phagocytosis, 34, 46, 50ff
phallotoxins, 112ff
phlebitis, 19, 28f, 39ff, 147
phlebology, 29, 147
phosphoglucomutase, 16
pigmentary retinities, 18
pituitary, 96ff
placebo effect, 100
platelet aggregation inhibition,
    17, 20, 65, 79, 128
polymerase, 95
polymerase A, 117
polysomes, 94f
post-operative recovery, 28
post-thrombotic syndrome, 29

p-oxyphenylpyruvic acid (OPH), 110
praseodymium, 114
pregnancy, 20, 37
presbyacusia, 72
proctitis, 29, 147
proctology, 29, 73f, 81, 147
properdin, 52, 54
prostacyclin, 132
prostaglandins, 54
protein, 116f, 136f
protein synthesis, 94f
proteolytic, 136
pruritus, 29, 147
pseudo-ephedrine, 11
p-tolymethylcarbinol, 130
punctate exudates, 28
purpuras, 147
ophthalmology, 17ff
quercetin, 12, 63, 66, 70, 139f, 148f
rabies, 46
radiation sickness, 102
radiation surgery, 38
radiation ulcers, 37
rare earths, 114
Raynaud's disease, 76
regeneration, cellular, 116ff, 120
reticulo-endothelial system, 34
retina, disease, 15ff, 148f
retinal hemorrhage, 20, 28f, 147
retinal lesions, 67
retinal purple, 15ff
retinitis, pigmentary, 18
retinopathy, diabetic, 28f, 147
rheumatism, 49
rhodopsin, 15ff
ribosomes, 95
ringing in ears, 72, 76, 80
RNA, 89, 94f, 101, 116f
rods, 15ff
rubella, 57
ruscogenins, 25ff
rutin, 12, 139
saponins, 25ff, 87ff, 94
schizophrenia, 33
sclerosis, 35ff, 77, 145
scopolamine, 11, 67
sedative, 20, 33, 90, 92, 101, 140